THE

HERPES

BOOK

THE
HERPES
BOOK

RICHARD HAMILTON, M.D.

J. P. Tarcher, Inc.
Los Angeles

Distributed by
Houghton Mifflin Company
Boston

The extract on page 105 is reprinted by permission
from *Getting Well Again,* by O. Carl Simonton, M.D.,
Stephanie Matthews-Simonton, and James Creighton.
Published by J. P. Tarcher, Inc., Los Angeles, 1978.

Design by John Brogna
Manufactured in the United States of America
Published by J.P. Tarcher, Inc.
9110 Sunset Blvd., Los Angeles, Calif. 90069
K10 9 8 7 6 5
First Edition

CONTENTS

INTRODUCTION

Even though herpes simplex virus disease (commonly referred to as just herpes) is one of the most prevalent viral diseases now known, to most infected people it brings only minimal discomfort. In its most usual form, the virus is responsible for the occasional and infrequent appearance of blisterlike sores on or around the lips. These lesions are called cold sores or fever blisters and, as most people who get them know, they are annoying and uncomfortable but rarely cause anguish, distress, or major medical difficulty. Left alone, the sores generally dry up and heal completely in about two weeks. The technical name for this form of the disease is labial herpes.

Over the past ten years or so, another form of the disease has been appearing with increasing frequency: genital herpes. As its name implies, it is a herpes infection, and it resembles cold sores in every way except one—it occurs on or around the sex organs. And although it is annoying and uncomfortable, it, too, rarely causes anguish, distress, or major medical difficulty and disappears by itself in about two weeks.

This brings up an important question. Why write a book about herpes, which, although widespread, is not usually considered troublesome or dangerous in either of its two major forms?

The answer is simple. Although the virus does not usually create problems for those who are infected, in a small percentage of cases it does, and in these cases its effects are pronounced, dramatic, far-reaching, and sometimes dangerous. It is mainly for the benefit of these people that this book was written—but not entirely. It was also written for those who may develop herpes at some future time and for the friends and relatives of people with herpes, who may be called upon for understanding, encouragement, support, and advice.

How can reading a book help people with a medical problem?

Herpes is no ordinary medical problem. Unlike infections caused by bacteria and other microbes against which penicillin, antibiotics, and other modern drugs are fully curative, herpes does not respond to any known form of therapy. Once a person is infected, the virus remains for life. Herpes cannot be cured, and this fact tends to shroud the other facts that are known about it. Having information that demystifies the nature of the infection, counteracts the myths and misinformation surrounding it, and provides a thorough understanding of what the virus is, what it does, and how the body responds to it fulfills a fundamental need of most people who experience a chronic condition—the need to know.

In addition to satisfying the basic need to understand what is going on, the information in this book has practical value in at least three other important areas: how to cope with the virus, how to prevent or minimize its possible complications, and how to distinguish fact from fiction in newspaper and magazine articles about the disease, which are appearing with increasing frequency.

Often the only difference between people who experience a terrible time with the virus and those who seem to cope and get along quite well is knowledge about how to manage the disease. For example, knowing that nutrition, sleep and rest, stress, general health, attitude, environmental factors, behavior, and hygiene may all affect the severity of the disease puts you in a position to exercise great influence over it.

Often the only difference between people who fall victim

to the complications of the disease and those who don't is an understanding of the risks and of the steps that may be taken either to prevent them entirely or to reduce them to near zero.

And often the only difference between people who needlessly waste energy and spend great sums of money for unsubstantiated or worthless "miracle cures"—only to have their hopes dashed when these cures fail to produce results—and those who aren't vulnerable to such claims is knowledge about the promising medical research that is now being carried out.

John F. Kennedy's often quoted phrase that knowledge is power just about says it all for people who want to gain personal mastery over this disease. I would add just one other observation: knowledge is hope. Knowledge that can be put to use in coping with herpes and knowledge that furnishes hope are what this book is all about.

I have attempted to arrange the material in this book in what I consider a logical progression, from the general to the specific, from the basic to the more complex. Accordingly, the first chapter answers the most frequently asked and basic questions about herpes. Except for the last chapter, which answers the more complicated questions that arise only when the fundamentals are understood, the balance of the book is devoted to expanding upon the concepts introduced in Chapter 1.

If you have herpes and after reading this book are less frightened, less in the dark, better able to cope, or more hopeful that progress toward a cure is being made, then the book will have succeeded. If you don't have herpes but after reading this book feel that you are in a better position to understand, encourage, and support those who do, then the book will also have succeeded. For despite its subject matter, this book isn't about illness and disease; it's about health.

—

CHAPTER 1

PREVIEW: THE MOST COMMONLY ASKED QUESTIONS ABOUT HERPES

—

WHAT IS HERPES?

Herpes is an infection in humans that generally affects mucous membranes or skin surfaces. The illness is caused by two closely related viruses: herpes simplex virus type 1 (HSV-1) and herpes simplex virus type 2 (HSV-2). Aside from differences that are important only to virologists, biochemists, microbiologists, and other medical researchers, the two types of herpes simplex viruses produce symptoms that are indistinguishable to the patient.

The outward signs of infection are blisterlike sores that appear on mucosal or skin surfaces such as the mouth, lips, face, abdomen, front genitals, anus, buttocks, or thighs. The site of infection generally corresponds to the location on the body where the virus enters.

Most people are familiar with the form of herpes that occurs on the face or lips or in the mouth. The popular terms cold sores and fever blisters are used to describe facial, labial, or oral forms of the infection. Less well known, although by no means rare, are the sores caused by the virus that occur below the waist, predominantly on the abdomen, genitals, or thighs. Studies indicate that infection below the waist is six to nine times less common than facial, labial, or oral infection.

Regardless of where on the body the infection is established, one attribute of the virus is constant: once inside the body, it never leaves. This is not to say that the infected person will experience sores continually or even intermittently. Most do not. It means that once having gained entry into the body, the virus cannot be expelled and will remain in some form, usually dormant, for the rest of the person's life.

SINCE SORES ON THE LIPS, FACE, OR GENITALS COULD BE SYMPTOMS OF OTHER ILLNESSES OR CONDITIONS, HOW CAN THEY BE DIAGNOSED AS HERPES?

The only way to find out whether or not sores are specifically caused by herpes is to see a doctor while the symptoms are present. And, as is pointed out in the question, since facial or genital sores can be the signs of many different conditions, including syphilis, scabies, chancroid, and superficial staph infection, most of which can be completely cured, having the sores diagnosed is very important.

The diagnosis of herpes can be made on the basis of the doctor's observation of the symptoms. Most physicians are able to arrive at an accurate determination merely by close inspection of the lesions and gathering background information about prior episodes—how the lesions developed, how long they lasted, and how they were manifested. The syndrome is so classical and well described in medical literature that clinical diagnosis is correct 95 percent of the time.

In those cases where examination and history alone are insufficient, several laboratory procedures may be employed to clarify ambiguities. Since the virus affects cells in a characteristic way, microscopic examination of cell samples taken from the sores is often helpful in the diagnosis. Blood tests have some value in that if they are negative it is an indication that the sores are not caused by herpes. Unfortunately, a positive blood test doesn't fully answer the question of what is causing the sore. By far the best test is a tissue culture, a relatively straightforward procedure in which a specimen of the fluid in the sore is placed in a culture system capable of supporting viral growth. The culture medium consists of living cells maintained at body temperature; if herpes grows in it, the test is conclusive and a positive diagnosis can be made. If proper procedures were followed, the failure of the virus to grow generally means that the sores from which the specimen was taken were not caused by herpes.

HOW WIDESPREAD IS HERPES?

Since doctors are not required by law to report how many cases of herpes they diagnose, nobody knows for sure how many people are infected. However, a number of medical surveys have been conducted to help define the scope of the problem, and on the basis of these reports scientists estimate that between 50 million and 150 million people in the United States alone are infected with labial and genital herpes.

This estimate certainly is impressive and points to a large problem, but don't be overly impressed by it: nobody is absolutely certain what it means. The surveys usually involve taking blood tests from various segments of the population and then extrapolating to the population as a whole. The problem with this procedure is that a positive blood test can't distinguish between someone with a true case of recurrent herpes and someone who contracted the virus, experienced a primary episode, and was never bothered again. A positive test can only reveal that at one time that person acquired the virus.

Additional approaches, such as direct patient surveys and evaluation of medical records, have been employed to give greater definition to the data, but, in general, the number of patients involved and the number of records evaluated have been so small that extrapolation to the entire population of the United States is not possible with any degree of accuracy.

If pressed, most researchers and scientists will concede that estimates about the magnitude of the herpes problem are based on sound clinical experience, well-ordered logic, and a good deal of medical intuition and insight.

The best, most educated guess about the prevalence of recurrent herpes is that no fewer than 5 million Americans experience the genital form of the disease and no fewer than 50 million experience the oral, lip, or facial form. Even if these estimates are high by as much as 50 percent, they still indicate a major epidemic of herpes.

HOW IS HERPES CONTRACTED?

Herpes simplex viruses are infectious agents. Furthermore, they are *contact* infectious agents. Unlike cold and influenza viruses, which are airborne in droplets expelled by coughs and sneezes, or other viruses that are carried by insects and animals, herpes simplex viruses can live only in humans and are spread from person to person directly, without any environmental or other intermediary agent. Simply put, people spread herpes simplex viruses to other people.

The virus can be spread in several different ways. Since the lips, mouth, and face are the most common sites of herpes infection, it is not surprising that the virus is most often transmitted by kissing. The disease is often contracted during childhood, in which case family members—mothers, fathers, siblings, and close relatives—are frequently the sources of infection.

The form of the disease that occurs below the waist is also spread in a direct manner, most often during sexual relations; genital herpes is rarely seen in patients who have not begun sexual activity. Studies conducted by the U.S. Public Health Service indicate that—unlike labial herpes, which is typically acquired before puberty—genital infection occurs with increasing frequency as young people progress from the teenage years to early adulthood (ages 20 to 29).

The virus requires neither an open break in the skin nor an orifice in order to enter the body. Mucous membranes and the soft skin around the genital area are sufficiently permeable to allow entry. Upon contact, the virus has little difficulty penetrating the surface cells and becoming established.

WHAT HAPPENS WHEN YOU BECOME INFECTED WITH THE VIRUS?

The disease follows a typical pattern of development in most people. Approximately two to twenty days after the virus enters the body, a single sore or cluster of sores with a fluid-filled or blisterlike appearance develops near or at the site of viral invasion. In persons who acquire the virus orally or facially, these sores usually appear in the mouth or on the lips, chin, cheeks, or the skin around the lips. In persons who are infected genitally, the sores usually develop on, around, or just inside the sex organs.

Regardless of location, external sores may burn, itch, or be quite painful. Their development may sometimes be accompanied by swollen lymph glands, general muscular aches, fever, and malaise (an overall sickly feeling). In addition, women whose sores are just inside the vagina occasionally experience either a burning sensation when urinating or a mild vaginal discharge, or both.

These sores generally last for two to three weeks, during which time they progressively diminish; the fluid becomes less evident and, gradually, scabbing begins to occur. Muscle aches and fever subside, and swollen glands begin to return to normal. By the end of the second week, new skin or mucosal tissue begins to cover the surface where the sore once appeared, marking the end of the primary episode.

Despite outward appearances, the conclusion that all is well again is not entirely warranted. Although the evidence of infection is no longer manifest, the virus has not been eradicated from the body; rather, it remains, in a dormant state, in nerve tissue near the site of infection. In the case of oral, labial, or facial herpes, the latent virus takes up residence in a nerve cluster called the trigeminal ganglion, located near the cheek bone. In the case of genital herpes, the virus lies dormant in the sacral ganglion, located outside the spinal canal.

The virus can remain dormant in these nerve cells for extended periods without causing any noticeable damage or difficulty. On occasion, however, and for reasons that are not well understood, it can emerge from its latent state and track along neural pathways back to skin or mucosal surfaces (usually close to the site of original infection) and create an active, recurrent infection. Recurrences resemble the primary episode, except that they tend to be less severe. They generally don't hurt as much, last as long, or cause such pronounced swelling of the lymph glands.

IS HERPES ALWAYS RECURRENT?

No. Even though infection with herpes simplex viruses brings with it the potential for recurrences, because the body never fully rids itself of all viral matter, not everyone experiences the recurrent form of the disease. The proportion of those who contract herpes, experience an initial episode, and are never bothered again is not known precisely but is estimated to be a quarter to a third of all cases. Furthermore, a large number of those infected—perhaps an additional one-third—may experience reactivation of the virus so infrequently as to cause them little concern. Only the remaining one-third of the patients may actually be identified as subject to periodic reappearances of active virus sores.

Not only is recurrent herpes confined to a minority of those infected, but it can also be highly variable. The virus may recur as seldom as once in several years or much more often, and with uncanny regularity—monthly, bi-monthly, or several times a year. Even among persons who clearly suffer from repeated attacks of the virus, the frequency and duration of recurrences may vary greatly over time. Many infected people experience regular patterns of reactivation for a number of years followed by long intervals during which the virus remains inactive. Sometimes the previous pattern reappears and sometimes it doesn't. At other times, active infection may recur, but with an altogether different pattern.

CAN AN INFECTED PERSON DO ANYTHING TO CONTROL RECURRENCES?

There are two important factors—general health and stress —that may be related to viral reactivation. Thus any attention given to maintaining good health and avoiding stress may help to lessen a pattern of frequent recurrence.

Since medical science has yet to develop a substance that is fully curative and completely safe in dealing with herpes, the body is largely on its own in limiting viral activity. General health maintenance, which includes a balanced diet, good nutrition, and adequate rest and sleep, can lead to heightened overall resistance to infection. When a person is in a state of good health, the body's natural defenses are well equipped to counter the virus, not only by limiting recurrences, but by diminishing their severity. When a person's health is not properly maintained, the body's natural defenses are weakened and lack the ability to check the virus; in these cases, recurrences may be more frequent and more severe.

In addition to focusing on factors that promote and maintain good general health, understanding the relationship between stress and susceptibility to illness is valuable, because —although its precise role has not been defined—stress is known to be involved in viral recurrence. Stress may directly trigger viral activity or, by lowering resistance, it may indirectly pave the way for a reemergence of the virus. Regardless of the exact manner in which stress may precipitate attacks, there is no doubt that it is a contributing factor.

DO ANY SPECIAL PRECAUTIONS HAVE TO BE TAKEN WHEN SORES ARE PRESENT?

During the active phase of herpes, three things have to be guarded against: secondary infection, spread of the virus to a new site on the body, and exposure of others to the virus.

Intact skin and mucous membranes form an important protective barrier against infection by many bacteria and microorganisms. When lesions develop because of herpes, they offer potential entry points for bacterial and other agents. These organisms can in turn cause a secondary infection on top of the herpes, and in some cases they can be many times more painful and distressing than the herpes itself. To minimize the risk of bacterial infection, herpes sores should be kept clean and, above all, dry; ointments and creams, except those prescribed to treat secondary infections, tend to prolong the lesions. To the greatest extent possible, avoid scratching, picking, rubbing, or touching the sores.

Each time herpes sores reappear, large numbers of viral particles are present at the site of infection. During these periods it is important not to transfer the virus to a new location on the body, a process known as autoinoculation. Several simple procedures will minimize the risk of accidental viral transfer. (1) Don't touch the sores. (2) Wash your hands if you inadvertently do touch the sores. (3) When you wake up, wash your hands *before* rubbing your eyes. (4) If you wear contact lenses and there are sores in your mouth or on your lips, don't use saliva as a wetting agent for the lenses. (Under no circumstances should you insert contact lenses without first washing your hands.) If you follow these rules, you will reduce the risk of transferring the virus to a new site, particularly to your eyes, which are quite vulnerable.

Finally, when sores are present you should be very careful not to spread the infection to others. During the entire period, such direct-contact activities as kissing and (in the case of genital-area lesions) sex should be avoided.

WHEN AND HOW CAN HERPES BE TRANSMITTED?

The consensus among physicians is that herpes can be transmitted only when viral particles are present at skin or mucosal surfaces. In general, this condition exists as long as sores are present, during either initial or recurrent attacks.

Herpes simplex viruses can be transmitted only by direct contact with the cells of an uninfected person. The invariables here are viral presence and direct contact. If either is missing, viral spread is highly unlikely. For instance, during the latent period when the virus is dormant in nerve tissue some distance from skin or mucosal surfaces, concern about transmission is unwarranted. Even when sores containing active viruses *are* present, if there is no direct contact by an uninfected person to the affected area there is no need to be concerned about spreading the infection.

These stringent requirements for transmission mean that even those relatively few people who experience frequently recurring sores need not worry about infecting someone else. They must avoid direct contact only for the short time they are actively infectious in order to prevent viral spread. And, of course, when the sores aren't present, the disease can't be transmitted at all.

CAN HERPES SIMPLEX VIRUS DISEASE BE PREVENTED?

Yes, but not in the way that other viral diseases are prevented. Polio, smallpox, measles, rubella, and influenza can be prevented by vaccination, which renders one immune regardless of exposure. There is as yet no such immunizing agent for herpes, and therefore the key to prevention is to eliminate exposure to the virus.

Behavioral intervention is a powerful technique to curb the spread of herpes. Unlike vaccination, however, which requires no forethought (once immunized, you are protected), behavioral intervention presupposes three things: (1) the knowledge that you are infected, (2) a firm understanding of when and how you are infectious to others, and (3) a conscious desire to do something about it. Assuming all three conditions are met, you are in an ideal position to prevent transmission of the virus.

Since the virus is transmissible only when lesions are present, those wishing not to spread it need only curtail direct contact during times of active outbreaks. This may mean no kissing or no sex (depending on the site of infection) for the interval of time commencing with onset and continuing through disappearance of lesions. Sores that occur internally make it somewhat more difficult to know when to refrain from direct contact with others, but even in these situations one can learn to recognize the subtle indications (such as internal tingles, itching, tenderness, and other signs that will be discussed later) of an active virus and prevent transmission in spite of not being able to see the sores.

IS HERPES CONSIDERED DANGEROUS?

Most cases of herpes are annoying, frustrating, bothersome, and inconvenient, but not dangerous. There are two circumstances when the disease is potentially threatening: if it is transmitted to the eyes or if it infects the brain. In addition, genital herpes in women may present some special problems. Before explaining these possible dangers, it is well to note that they are quite rare, almost always preventable, and almost always treatable.

The eyes are especially vulnerable to infection, and if the virus is introduced into an eye it can cause lesions on the cornea, which may result in partial or complete vision impairment. This condition is known as herpes keratitis. Fortunately, the eyes are rarely the site of initial infection; most often they are affected as the result of autoinoculation, which can usually be prevented. In rare cases the virus can travel directly from the trigeminal ganglion to the eye, but even when the virus does infect the eyes, new antiviral drugs such as ara-A and IDU can prevent damage if the condition is treated in time.

Herpes encephalitis is the complication that occurs if the brain becomes infected. This is extremely rare, however, and occurs only when a virus present at sites on the face or lips or in the mouth travels to the brain along nerve pathways from the trigeminal ganglion. Fortunately, not only is herpes encephalitis rare, but, like herpes keratitis, it can also be treated.

There are two potential problems associated with genital herpes in women: the possible (though yet unproven) link with cervical cancer and the risk of passing the virus to a baby during birth. Both potential dangers can be prevented by simple precautions. Regular PAP tests can detect changes in cervical tissue long before an actual cancer develops, at an early enough stage so that the problem can be dealt with effectively. And if an obstetrician is informed about a pregnant woman's history of recurrent genital herpes, simple steps can be taken to minimize the possibility that the baby will be infected during birth.

HOW RELEVANT IS THE PRESENCE OF GENITAL HERPES IN WOMEN TO THE DEVELOPMENT OF CERVICAL CANCER?

Research indicates that there is an association between the two, but it is important to keep in mind that no cause-and-effect relationship has been proven. Genital herpes is not considered a precursor of cervical cancer; it simply is one of several factors correlated with increased risk.

The association between genital herpes in women and increased risk of cervical cancer is based on three factors. First, statistical observation reveals that women with genital herpes more frequently develop cervical cancer and cancer-like changes in cervical tissue than women who don't have genital herpes. Second, medical researchers have found that some test animals infected with the virus subsequently developed cancer at or near the site of the infection. Third, fragments of the virus have been found in the abnormal cells obtained from women with cervical cancer.

Again, it is important to bear in mind that association is not causation. Certainly not all women with genital herpes develop cervical cancer; very few do. But, in relative terms, more women who have genital herpes subsequently develop such a cancer than do women who are not subject to herpes.

Knowing that genital herpes is viewed as a factor of increased risk, however, women who are infected should take appropriate precautions to protect themselves. Having a PAP test at least once a year, and possibly every six months, can help reduce and almost eliminate the risk of invasive cervical cancer. Cell changes that are detected early by a

PAP test can almost always be treated easily and completely, usually right in the doctor's office.

In general, the association between genital herpes and cervical cancer should be more an impetus to simple and appropriate preventive action than a cause for undue worry and concern.

CAN WOMEN WITH GENITAL HERPES HAVE BABIES?

The answer is an unqualified yes. Not only can they, but women with genital herpes are giving birth to healthy babies all the time. The key to coping successfully with this condition during pregnancy is to be aware of the problem and share your awareness with your obstetrician.

Since the major risk of exposure and transmission occurs around the time of delivery, an obstetrician who has been alerted in advance can closely monitor the condition of the birth canal during the last several weeks of gestation. If active lesions are noted and the risk to the baby is considered great, the obstetrician may choose to deliver the baby by Caesarean section rather than chance a normal delivery during which exposure might occur. If, upon examination, there is no evidence of viral activity in the birth canal, there is no risk of exposing the baby, and normal delivery may be chosen.

CAN HERPES BE TREATED?

The answer is a qualified yes. As already stated, herpes keratitis and herpes encephalitis, if caught early enough, can be treated effectively with new drugs designed to halt the progress of the virus in the eyes and in the brain. As far as surface lesions are concerned, no such therapies exist as yet (the drugs used for eye and brain infections were tried on surface sores but did not work).

Even though the progress of the virus in surface sores cannot be halted by any drugs presently available, there are a variety of drugs and preparations a doctor may prescribe to lessen the pain, burning, itching, or other discomfort that may accompany lesions. There are also several agents that may help bolster the natural healing process, as well as antibacterial creams and ointments with which to treat secondary infections.

The search for curative antiviral compounds that are effective against recurrent herpes is an exciting and important area of research in which many university medical centers and a number of commercial pharmaceutical firms are engaged. At the present time, several promising antiviral agents are at various stages of development and testing. None is commercially available yet, but the consensus is that the day when herpes can be controlled, and possibly cured, is not far in the future.

CHAPTER 2

THE HISTORY
OF HERPES

A FAMILY OF VIRUSES

We have been using the terms *virus* and *herpes* rather loosely. Here we will be more precise and add some definition to them, enough for a more thorough understanding of the material in this chapter.

To begin with, viruses are much smaller than bacteria. If you have ever seen a photograph of a bacterium or examined one firsthand in a high school or college biology class, you know that what you are seeing has been magnified hundreds, and sometimes thousands, of times. If you consider that there is enough room inside the body of this microscopic organism to comfortably contain hundreds of thousands, and perhaps millions, of viruses—that's small.

Next, viruses aren't alive. When you examine bacteria through the eyepiece of a microscope, what you see is fascinating. There is movement and activity. You can watch them eat, eliminate wastes, and—if you wait long enough—reproduce themselves by dividing. When you look at a virus, however, what you see is dull, stagnant, unanimated. There is no movement, no eating, no waste elimination, no division; in short, there are none of the attributes of life.

Finally, viruses are invasive intracellular parasites. This is not as complicated as it sounds. Let's compare viruses with bacteria again. Bacteria are also parasites, in that when they enter the body of a host they satisfy their need for fluids and nutrients by competing with cells for available supplies. Viruses, however, have no such need because they aren't alive. Instead, viruses enter cells and stay there. Sometimes their presence damages the cell so greatly that it no longer provides suitable refuge, and then the viruses simply invade a nearby cell and take up residence there.

Obviously, there is a lot more to say about viruses, and we will later, but for now it is sufficient to know that viruses are infinitesimally small, nonliving parasites that invade cells. All viruses work essentially the same way, including the group of viruses in which we are interested, the herpesviruses.

Like animals, plants, and even bacteria, viruses are classified into family groups and subgroups according to their similarities. The broadest category is "family," and that's what herpes is—the family name for over fifty related viruses that share certain common characteristics: similar size, shape, structure, and internal composition. But there are differences, and the differences give rise to the subgroups.

Some herpesviruses infect only oysters, and they constitute one subgroup. Others are limited to chickens, turkeys, frogs, mice, squirrels, monkeys, rabbits, and even fungi, each constituting a separate, species-specific subgroup. The subgroup that infects people comprises five different herpesviruses.

The best-known human herpesvirus is the varicella-zoster (VZ) virus, which causes the common childhood disease chickenpox and another infection in adults called shingles (technically known as herpes zoster). And who hasn't heard of mono? Infectious mononucleosis is caused principally by another human herpesvirus called the Epstein-Barr virus (EBV). Not as well known as chickenpox, shingles, or infectious mononucleosis is an infant infection called cytomegalic inclusion disease, which, as it turns out, is caused by yet another human herpesvirus, the cytomegalovirus (CMV). Finally, there are the two remaining human herpesviruses, herpes simplex virus type 1 (HSV-1) and type 2 (HSV-2).

These are the closely related culprits that cause labial and genital herpes.

Because the minor differences between HSV-1 and HSV-2 are of no particular importance to patients, or even to most doctors (they are only important to molecular microbiologists, virologists, and other researchers), and because our only concern is with herpes simplex virus disease, we can drop all distinctions and simply refer to the disease as herpes. Where our discussions require more specificity, I will furnish it.

HERPES AND HUMANITY: A TWO-THOUSAND-YEAR RELATIONSHIP

There are many theories that seek to explain how viruses originated, and, specifically, how herpesviruses developed. Some suggest that they preceded life, others that they evolved concomitantly with life. The most plausible theory is that viruses came after life, originating as elements of normal cells that acquired a form of incomplete autonomy. This is certainly consistent with their intimate association with cells and their specificity to individual species (frog herpesviruses never infect humans, and vice versa), although it's just theoretical speculation.

If the origin of herpesviruses is somewhat uncertain and obscure, their long-standing relationship to humanity is not. Herpes simplex viruses have been with us a long time. They can, in fact, be counted among our most lasting legacies from the past.

The ancient Greeks knew about herpes. Their physicians studied the disease, wrote about it, and gave it a name. The word *herpes,* from the Greek word meaning "to creep," described what the Greeks were observing—sores that seemed to creep over the surface of the skin.

The ancient Romans knew about herpes as well. Nearly two thousand years ago, Roman Emperor Tiberius attempted to curb an epidemic of herpes labialis by outlawing kissing at public ceremonies and rituals.

Over the next nineteen hundred years, physicians in every

civilized society continued to chronicle their experiences with herpes much as the early Greeks and Romans had done. In 1886, two French physicians, Diday and Doyon, published the first comprehensive medical review of the genital form of the disease. Ten years later, in 1896, a German physician named Unna published a clinical review that covered herpes labialis as well. In 1921, Dr. B. Lipschütz, also of Germany, wrote what at the time was the most complete medical review of herpes ever published. This was an amazing accomplishment, for although viruses—or, more accurately, things smaller than bacteria—were known to exist, they still had never been seen and their nature had not yet been defined. Dr. Lipschütz was able to attribute—prophetically—herpes labialis and herpes genitalis to different viruses, a fact that wasn't to be proven until over forty years later.

Many people wonder how viruses could have been studied in the late-nineteenth and early-twentieth centuries, several decades before the development of the powerful microscopes, computer-monitored lab equipment, and other modern tools that are used today. The answer is a credit to the value of both descriptive medicine, a discipline dating back thousands of years, and medical sleuthmanship—deductive reasoning applied to reported observations.

The earliest discoveries about viruses were made in the last decade of the nineteenth century as a result of studying a well-described disease of tobacco plants, tobacco mosaic disease (so called because of the mosaiclike lesions that occurred on the leaves of sick plants). In 1892, scientists conclusively proved that the disease was caused by an infectious agent that was different from any bacteria known at the time.

They found that extracts of diseased leaves applied to healthy plants caused the healthy plants to become sick and develop lesions; however, when the extracts were viewed under the most powerful microscopes of the time—microscopes capable of detecting bacteria—no organisms were visible. From this the researchers concluded that the infectious agent had to be smaller than 1/125,000 of an inch.

Their small size was confirmed by scientists in another manner. When the extract was passed through earthenware filters with pores small enough to trap bacteria, the infectious agent emerged on the other side.

A further difference was noted between this still-invisible agent and bacteria: it could not be cultured using any of the standard media or processes that were used reliably to grow bacteria artificially, but seemed dependent on a living host, the tobacco plant, in order to multiply.

Not knowing what else to call it (they were convinced, and rightly so, that it wasn't a bacterium, for it defied every known property of bacteria), they devised the term *virus*, from the Latin word for "poison," to describe the agents that caused tobacco mosaic disease and such other illnesses as hoof-and-mouth disease in cattle (attributed to a virus in 1898) and yellow fever in humans (attributed to a virus in 1901). The term was applied to all agents that seemed to share the properties not only of extreme smallness but, even more important, of being able to reproduce only in living hosts.

In those early years of viral study, scientists were hampered by their inability to grow viruses, including herpes simplex viruses, and their work remained more descriptive than experimental.

In the late 1920s and early 1930s, when new methods were devised for working with and studying not only herpes simplex viruses but all viruses, purely descriptive science began to yield to experimentation accompanied by an expansion in the development of insight and information.

New filters of known-average-pore diameter were developed. Many times more precise than the earlier earthenware filters, they permitted an accurate estimate of the size of different viruses, including herpes.

Then, convenient experimental animal models were introduced when scientists devised ways of artificially infecting rabbits. Once they were able to study how the virus progressed, destroyed tissue, and traveled along nerve pathways, researchers were able to learn about and record the natural history of herpes in a comprehensive and controlled manner. Some of the earliest insights into herpes encephalitis (infection of the brain), herpes keratitis (infection of the eye), and neonatal herpes (infection of newborns) resulted from this work with lab animals.

By the middle 1930s, when the relatively young science of virology was firmly established and developing rapidly, a stunning technological advancement captured the imagination of scientists and laypersons alike, enabling them to see sights that had never before been seen. With the electron microscope, scientists could peer into a world so infinitely small that new terms had to be invented to describe it. Using this marvelous new invention, which focuses and then electronically amplifies beams of electrons instead of visible rays of light, for the first time scientists were able to come face to face with humankind's smallest enemies, whose existence up to that point had been known only by the diseases they caused.

Great numbers of viruses were studied now that their sizes, shapes, and structures were plainly visible. On the basis of these physical characteristics, groupings were made and families of viruses identified. Herpesviruses, for instance, were found to be large in relation to other viruses, highly complex in structure, and surrounded by what appeared to be a protective envelope.

The earliest theories about the nature of viruses were finally confirmed by direct microscopic examination. By themselves, viruses were found to be inert, displaying none of the attributes of bacteria or other microorganisms: they possessed no mobility of their own; they didn't seem to require nourishment; they didn't eliminate waste (understandably, since there was no waste to eliminate); they didn't even reproduce, the most essential activity of organisms. They seemed to be totally dependent on the host; once inside, their apparent lifelessness was replaced by enormous levels of activity. Within the host, they behaved just like bacteria —with one important difference.

Unlike bacteria, which are capable of carrying on their life functions just about anywhere in the body—on the surface of skin, in the bloodstream, and in the space between cells— viruses were found to "live" actively in only one environment: inside an invaded cell. It appeared that viruses were incomplete by themselves, entirely dependent on the machinery of a cell to express lifelike functions. It was as though they were pure information, possessing the knowledge of how to do something—move, metabolize, reproduce—but lacking the independent means to do so. As further viral study would reveal, nothing could have been closer to the truth.

There was a problem, however, in the pursuit of more information. As marvelous as they were, electron microscopes were useless without specimens of the virus to examine, and in that early age of viral discovery the demand for specimens far outstripped supply. The problem of growing the virus artificially to provide sufficient samples for more extensive and intensive study was a hurdle that simply had to be overcome if progress were to continue.

The breakthrough came in 1949, when cell-culture systems were developed. These systems consist of cells maintained in a living state into which viruses are introduced and which thereafter can be observed or harvested. Although less spectacular than the invention of the electron microscope, cell-culture technology represented an innovation that was equally as important, if not more so. Scientists could now artificially grow and harvest large numbers of viruses for study and experimentation. In addition, scientists could recreate and witness the cell-disrupting effects of viruses under highly controlled laboratory conditions.

Soon thereafter, in 1953, virus-research scientists devised a method for measuring the cell-disrupting and cell-killing effects of viruses. By introducing a known quantity of viruses onto a single layer of cells and counting the holes in the cell layer caused by the viruses, they could determine the virulence of the virus. This standard test is still in use today.

Now investigators could not only see and grow the virus, but they could also study and quantify its ability to disrupt the function of invaded cells. From this point on, progress in viral research moved at an ever-increasing rate.

Techniques were perfected to purify viruses—that is, to separate them from the cells in which they grew—which made it easier to study them. Interactions between viruses and cells were observed, and this led to the development of tests that could detect these interactions. Since viruses were too small to take apart using mechanical means, chemical and physical-chemical dissection methods were devised. Every aspect, every property, every component of the virus came under close scrutiny, and an entirely new vocabulary had to be developed to describe what was learned.

By 1960, the herpes simplex virus and herpes simplex virus disease had been well characterized and closely examined. A number of complications affecting the brain, eyes, and newborn babies had been extensively studied, as had the mechanism by which the virus disrupts cells. It was beginning to seem as though scientists had taken descriptive and analytical processes as far as they could when another major breakthrough added an entirely new dimension to herpes research and became the starting point for a new wave of scientific interest in the virus.

Between 1961 and 1968, investigators in Germany and the United States were finding that herpes simplex virus disease was caused not by one virus but by two closely related, though differentiable, viruses. Because these viruses were so similar, both were still called herpes simplex, their minor differences being denoted by the addition of type 1 or type 2.

The distinction between herpes simplex virus type 1 (HSV-1) and type 2 (HSV-2) was made on the basis of several factors, most of them technical (molecular composition, growth patterns in cell cultures, and different antibodies elicited by each), though one—a clinical difference—was profoundly interesting in its human implications and still remains one of the more fascinating features of herpes simplex virus disease.

Forty years earlier, Dr. Lipschütz had suggested that herpes labialis and herpes genitalis, although appearing to be identical in all regards except for the site of infection, might be attributed to different viruses. He turned out to have been absolutely correct. When the techniques to differentiate the virus types were developed in the mid-1960s, scientists found that nearly all cases of herpes labialis were caused by

HSV-1, while nearly all cases of herpes genitalis were caused by HSV-2.

Why was this so? Could these almost identical viruses possess an undiscovered major difference in the kind of tissue for which they had an affinity? This theory was rejected, because in a small percentage of cases HSV-1 was found to cause genital infection and HSV-2 to cause infections on the lips. The tissue type didn't seem to matter to either of the viruses.

The answer turned out to be a simple matter of human behavior. For whatever reason, thousands—perhaps tens of thousands—of years ago, HSV-1 had emerged as the agent that caused sores around the lips. Similarly, in years past and for whatever reason, HSV-2 had emerged as the agent that caused genital infection. Since both forms of the virus are transmitted in the same way, by direct contact, the only logical conclusion was that oral-genital sexual contact remained a highly limited practice over thousands of years and in countless different cultures.

Is there any evidence to support this conclusion? In a sense there is. In the mid-1960s, it became technologically possible to distinguish between HSV-1 and HSV-2, the virus types were isolated from unexpected sites (HSV-2 from lip sores and HSV-1 from genital sores) in approximately 5 percent of cases. Today, in the so-called sexual-revolution years; the number of cases in which the virus types are cultured from unexpected sites has jumped to between 10 and 15 percent.

In a roundabout way, this increased proportion of lip herpes caused by HSV-2 and genital herpes caused by HSV-1 could be taken to mean that oral-genital sexual practices are more commonplace today. An alternative possibility is that enough cases of HSV-2–caused lip sores and HSV-1–caused genital sores exist to ensure continued spread to these unlikely sites in the usual manners—that is, by kissing and sexual intercourse. The likelihood is that both factors have contributed to the current finding and will continue to do so. It is entirely possible that years from now these two virus types will lose their site-specific characteristics, and the chances of finding HSV-1 or HSV-2 in any case of herpes will be 50-50.

The discovery that there were two naturally occurring

variants of the herpes simplex virus not only provoked renewed interest among researchers but allowed public-health officials and epidemiologists to begin to investigate the magnitude and public-health dimension of herpes. By employing the blood test used to detect and differentiate antibodies to HSV-1 and HSV-2, whole populations could be surveyed by a process called seroepidemiologic study to gauge prevalence, spread patterns, risk factors, and consequences. (We will cover antibodies in greater detail later; to understand this chapter it is sufficient to know that our bodies produce antibodies against foreign organisms and that these antibodies can be detected in the blood.)

Some of the earliest seroepidemiologic studies were conducted by the research groups most active in herpes investigations, those at the Emory University School of Medicine in Atlanta, the Baylor College of Medicine in Houston, and the University of Washington School of Medicine in Seattle. Dr. E. R. Alexander of the University of Washington studied HSV-1 antibody levels in people from different socioeconomic groups and found that in families of modest means antibodies to HSV-1 could be detected in the blood of nearly all children by the time they were 5 years old. This was not the case among children coming from affluent homes. Antibodies to HSV-1 were rarely detected among these youngsters; the count rose to only 30 percent of people by the time they reached 20. By far the most interesting finding, however, was that by the time people turned 50 the socioeconomic differences had disappeared and nearly everyone had HSV-1 antibodies in their blood. The differences noted among children and younger people could easily be explained by cultural variations in how openly family affection is expressed and how entrenched herpes is in a group to begin with.

Dr. Andre Nahmias, a pioneer in herpes research at Emory University, conducted a similar study among people from different socioeconomic backgrounds, testing for HSV-2 antibody levels. He detected HSV-2 antibodies in 10 percent of adults from higher socioeconomic groups as compared to between 20 and 60 percent of adults from less affluent backgrounds. Here again, the relative degree to which the disease was already entrenched among the groups as well as cultural variations in sexual mores tend to explain these differences.

Dr. Joseph Melnick and Dr. W. E. Rawls of Baylor conducted a study of a different nature. They went looking for HSV-2 antibodies in two highly diverse groups of people—prostitutes and nuns. Predictably (since HSV-2 is the frequent cause of genital herpes), they found that HSV-2 antibodies could be demonstrated in a large percentage of prostitutes and that the number climbed to nearly 100 percent as they got older. Among nuns, the HSV-2 antibody was rarely detected.

What do the findings of these seroepidemiologic studies indicate? First, they indicate a large and diverse problem. Since the presence of an antibody generally means that some encounter with one of the viruses has occurred, and since the HSV-1 or HSV-2 antibody is detectable in nearly all adults by the time they are 50 (mainly HSV-1), most scientists and public-health officials conclude that these viruses are extremely widespread in the population, and most agree with estimates that between one-third and two-thirds of the U.S. population has been infected with one of the viruses, approximately 10 percent of which is thought to be herpes simplex virus type 2.

Translated into numbers, this means that between 75 and 150 million Americans have been infected with HSV-1 or HSV-2. Although, fortunately, not everyone experiences recurrent herpes, enough do—approximately one-third—to classify herpes as the most prevalent, potentially serious communicable disease in the nation.

Second, the studies point compellingly to the need for prevention. Since there is no question that herpes is infectious, every person who experiences recurrence is potentially capable of transmitting the disease. And since the virus persists in the body forever, the value of prevention is all the more important, because prevention is the only effective way to cap this growing epidemic. Following is a description of what has happened—and will continue to happen unless the spread of herpes is curtailed.

Whatever the exact number, the present base of those infected with herpes is enormous, almost too large to imagine. It didn't develop overnight but evolved in much the same methodical way that other epidemic concentrations grow—person A gave it to person B, who in turn gave it to person C, and so on—with two major differences. Unlike most other infectious diseases, which may be cured with drugs or clear up by themselves, the virus that causes herpes remains in the body. And unlike most other infections that are communicable only for a limited, and usually brief, period, herpes is infectious during each recurrence. Both factors contribute to a more energetic and expansive epidemic growth pattern. Person A may give it to person B this month, to person C next year, to person D three years hence, and so on; and, of course, the pattern is repeated with persons B, C, and D.

Since each new person with recurrent herpes is able to infect any number of others, the unchecked epidemic will grow in a geometric fashion, continually broadening its base and growing ever more rapidly.

This risk of contracting the disease, therefore, is in direct proportion to its prevalence and the frequency with which carriers experience recurrences. In the absence of any way to diminish the present prevalence factor (those who have it, have it) or reliably limit recurrences, prevention of further spread is the one hope for stopping the epidemic.

The practice of prevention in cases of herpes boils down to one simple and highly effective rule: From the moment sores appear until the time they have healed completely, direct contact should be avoided. In the case of lip sores, this means no kissing; in the case of genital sores, it means no sex. Although abstaining from such fundamental human activities as kissing and sex, even for the limited time that sores are present, may at times be inconvenient and possibly awkward, there are no better options for reducing the risk to others. Considering its effectiveness and benefits, prevention makes a great deal of sense.

A relatively new concern about the potential consequences attributed to herpes arose from the early sero-epidemiologic studies to profile the disease, a public-health concern that had not existed before it was realized that herpes was so widespread. For although it is usually benign and self-limiting, as we have already noted, herpes can develop into more complicated and serious conditions, including encephalitis, keratitis, infection of newborns, and cervical cancer. And while the likelihood that any person might develop such a complication was still rare, the new knowledge that so many people were infected caused some worry that the frequency of complications in the entire population could rise in future years.

As a result, researchers and public-health officials, who had previously confined their writings and observations to scientific publications and medical journals, began to voice their concerns openly and become available for comment in the media. Between 1965 and 1975, dozens and dozens of newspaper and magazine articles about herpes appeared, and for the first time the public was being informed about a disease whose proportions and potential seriousness had never been fully appreciated.

In my opinion, this was good and very appropriate. There were a certain number of alarmist and sensational stories, but not many; most accounts stuck to the facts and told the story accurately and helpfully. Prevention was stressed, a theme so important, in my estimation, that you will see it repeated throughout this book. So was the emerging association of genital herpes with cervical cancer and, more important, the need for infected women to take frequent and regular PAP tests to minimize their risks. The potential tragedy of infant herpes was brought out, but so were the many things that informed women and knowledgeable doctors could do together to prevent it.

Yes, all the public exposure herpes received in those ten years—more than in the preceding two thousand—was good. Why avoid an issue because it might be unpleasant or upsetting when it makes greater sense to be informed about the risks and what can be done to counter them? Why leave such important matters to chance when, with information and heightened awareness, the odds can be influenced to the better?

There was one additional benefit derived from this new public interest: herpes research took on additional importance. Sensing a climate of concern and receptivity, established virologists, immunologists, and other scientists whose focus had been in other areas began to move into herpes research. At the same time, a young, new cadre of investigators with fresh ideas and novel approaches entered the field, and the work of these researchers at universities and medical schools throughout the country began to be financed by government grants at unprecedented levels. Hundreds of thousands of dollars were allocated rather than the much smaller sums of the past. And, finally, appreciating the commercial possibilities of safe and effective antiviral drugs, major pharmaceutical firms began to divert research-and-development resources into this important area of scientific pursuit. With so much interest being expressed by all sectors of society— academia, government, and industry—the question is no longer whether the problem can be solved, but when it will be solved.

Since ancient times, physicians and scientists have been documenting and describing a two-thousand-year relationship between humanity and two of its most tenacious and successful viral parasites, HSV-1 and HSV-2. For most of those two thousand years, doctors were relatively helpless to intercede or improve things because there were so few opportunities to do so. Today the opportunities are limitless. As we will see in the next chapter, herpes is a formidable foe, but so is the awesome natural defense our bodies can mount against it. And as we will see throughout this book, the opportunities are abundant for people with herpes to live without impediment and to the fullest.

CHAPTER 3

VIRUS VERSUS HOST, HOST VERSUS VIRUS

THE OUTWARD SIGNS

The first sign of herpes that most people notice is a tingling, itching, or burning sensation near the site of the developing infection. The surface sometimes appears slightly discolored and is almost invariably sensitive to touch. Within hours of the first tingling sensation, although occasionally a day or two may pass, one or more small red marks will appear on the affected surface. These marks may resemble a measles rash, but they are confined to a very small area, usually no wider than half an inch across. In a very short time, rarely more than a few hours, the small red marks develop into fluid-filled, blisterlike sores that appear watery and grayish at the center and red around the edges. The entire area near the sores may be swollen and inflamed, and the pain may be quite sharp, radiating outward to adjacent areas.

By this point, many people will be experiencing more general symptoms, the most common of which are swollen lymph glands, muscle aches, malaise (an overall sickly feeling), and fever.

Over the next two to ten days the fluid-filled sores will gradually perforate and begin to "weep." Before a scab forms, the weeping sores may appear to be punched-out or ulcerlike.

Scab formation generally marks a turning point in both the way the sores look and the way the affected person feels. Local swelling, inflammation, and pain begin to subside, and general symptoms start to diminish. The scabbed-over sores now look more like a healing cut than anything else. As new mucous membrane or skin develops, the scabs fall off and, generally, by the end of the second week most patients are almost completely recovered—or so it may appear.

HERPES AND FOOTBALL: AN ANALOGY

Football is an engrossing and dramatic sequence of events. The scoreboard, while an important recording device, merely hints at the excitement on the field, where the players are engaging in a competitive struggle for supremacy.

What does football have to do with herpes? Nothing really, except by way of analogy. The scoreboard—the outward signs described above—only reflects the far more dynamic sequence of events taking place on a playing field beneath the skin's surface. This playing field, of course, is the network of cells, tissue, capillaries, and lymph glands, a field marked off not in yards but in microns, roughly 100 million times smaller than a football field.

On the defensive line we have cellular components (specialized white blood cells) and chemical components (interferon, antibodies, lymphokines, and complements)—as swift and punishing a defense as any. For the offense (the analogy begins to fall apart somewhat here) there's only one player, the virus. The analogy breaks down completely concerning the rules of play, for there are none, or, rather, there is just one—survival.

Before taking a look at the struggle itself, let's get acquainted with all the principals who will participate: first the viral challenger, then the body's defense.

The Offense

Like all viruses, herpes simplex viruses are extremely small. They are in fact among the smallest disease-causing agents in nature, measuring only 8 millionths of an inch across. When compared to most other nonviral microbes—for example, bacteria and protozoa—herpes simplex viruses would seem like dwarfs, ranging from several to several hundred *times* smaller. When compared to other viruses, however, such as those causing the common cold, influenza, and yellow fever, herpes simplex is a relative giant.

But, for a virus, the herpes simplex virus is relatively fragile. While many microorganisms are well suited to survive exposure to the outside world by developing protective casings that insulate them from environmental factors such as light, heat, cold, and dryness, the herpes simplex virus cannot withstand such rigors. After only a few hours outside its milieu, the human body, it decomposes and simply ceases to exist. This is why inanimate objects are rarely involved in the transmission of herpes.

In addition to being many times smaller and unable to survive in the outside world, herpes simplex viruses differ from all other nonviral microscopic agents in a most important way: they are not alive. In fact, all viruses are nonliving microorganisms. Unlike bacteria and protozoa, which take in and metabolize food, give off waste products, move about, and, most fundamentally, reproduce—all essential aspects of the definition of life—viruses do none of these. How, then, do they continue to exist and, from time to time, create trouble?

Although lacking the ability to carry on life processes by themselves, all viruses, including herpes, are endowed with special chemical properties that enable them to move into a living cell and take over. They can force it to ignore its own life-support functions (which is damaging to the cell, to say the least) and, instead, expend all of its energy producing exact copies of more viruses. By definition, viruses are "obligate, intracellular parasites," meaning that they are obliged to depend on the cells they infect for continued existence and propagation. They are opportunists of the first order;

they do nothing for themselves, but they see to it that their needs are provided for by the cells they commandeer.

All of this power emanates from their genes. Viruses are almost pure genetic information and little else. These genes contain sets of instructions that, when activated in a living cell, subvert the normal genes of that cell and cause it to come under the total domination of the virus.

One last point about the viral challenger. Like any good offense, herpes simplex viruses not only possess the driving power and brute force to scuttle any but the best defense and press forward, but they also have the good sense to break off the attack when they are outclassed by a superior force of defenders. In this struggle, where the only prize is continued existence, retreat to a more defensible position is a sound survival strategy and one that is most cleverly accomplished by herpes simplex viruses. Once they enter nerve cells near the infection site, they may become inactive, and as long as they remain latent they are shielded from attack; as far as the defense is concerned, they no longer exist. But, as we will find out, retreat is not necessarily defeat.

In evolutionary terms, herpes simplex viruses are among our most worthy opponents. Their continued existence underscores this fact because, as we are about to see, the various cells and chemicals that make up the defense render the human body one of the most hostile environments in which to attempt survival.

The Defense

The defensive line consists in part of several specialized white blood cells: macrophages, B-lymphocytes, plasma cells, and T-lymphocytes. They all originate from bone marrow as primitive undifferentiated cells. Depending upon where they mature in the body, they take on individual characteristics and special functions. Their names may reflect their site of maturation, their special characteristics, or their function.

Macrophages not only originate in bone marrow but mature there as well. When they are released into the bloodstream they are ready to devour and digest prey. They take their name from the Greek words for large, *macro,* and eating, *phagein.*

B-lymphocytes are thought to undergo development and maturation in regions of the lymph system at either end of the intestinal tract. In birds, where B-lymphocytes were first recognized, they mature in an intestinal lymph organ known as the bursa, which is why they are designated as B.

Although most wait in readiness in the lymph nodes, a small number of B-lymphocytes continually circulate throughout our bodies, moving back and forth between the lymph and blood systems. Should they encounter a free-floating foreign invader or—in the case of HSV-1 or HSV-2—a cell that shows evidence of invasion, B-lymphocytes will pick up the defense by immediately cloning themselves (dividing into exact duplicates). Some of these clones will act as messengers by traveling to the nearest lymph node with chemical word of the invasion. Others will remain at the site of infection and transform into yet another kind of defensive cell, a plasma cell.

Plasma cells are transformed B-lymphocytes that produce and secrete special chemicals—antibodies—to fight foreign invaders. These antibodies coat the surface of invaders—or, in the case of herpes, the invaded cells—with a substance that attracts devouring macrophages and inspires them to greater defensive activity. The antibody coat also marks the invader for attack by another defensive component, the complement system. In addition to their role in the present battle, antibodies will remain long after the fight has ended and will serve as an early warning system in the event of future attack.

When the B-lymphocytes acting as messengers carry word of the invasion back to nearby lymph nodes, they not only marshal B-lymphocyte reinforcements but also summon another category of defensive cells, *T-lymphocytes.* These T-cells, so called because they mature in the thymus, a tiny gland in the neck, react to word of the invasion by heading directly for the site of infection.

The defensive action of T-lymphocytes is direct, brutal, and of particular importance in herpes. A T-lymphocyte that has been drawn into battle is converted into a specially equipped cell called a *lymphoblast* and immediately releases a number of different chemicals called *lymphokines.* One of these lymphokines, the macrophage activation factor (maf), incites macrophages to a state of digestive frenzy. Another, the migration inhibition factor (mif), prevents the frenzied macrophages from moving away from the site of infection. A third, lymphocyte transformation factor (tf), converts any nonparticipating T-cells into committed defenders. As part of their general defensive activity, some T-lymphocytes undergo a different transformation, becoming killer cells capable of producing a poison called *lymphotoxin* that is deadly to cells invaded by HSV-1 or HSV-2.

So much for the cellular components of the defense. Now let's take a look at the strictly chemical components that round it out. (You may have noticed that I have begun to use martial terms in my explanations. It can't be helped, for the defense mechanism of the body is warlike in many of its protective processes.)

The *complement system* is made up of nine individual proteins floating freely in the blood, designated C_1 through C_9, which acting together form a kind of explosive that is lethal both to invading foreign objects and the cells harboring them. The complement system works in conjunction with B-lymphocytes. As already noted, some B-lymphocytes transform into plasma cells that produce antibodies. These antibodies coat foreign objects and infected cells and mark them for attack by providing a perfect molecular groove into which C_1, the first component of the complement system, can fit. The ensuing chain reaction is both precise and deadly. Once in place on the surface of the foreign object or infected cell, C_1 provides a binding site for C_2, which in turn allows C_3 to bind, and so on. Each initiates binding by its successor until all nine components are bound. At that instant the components of the bomb are in place, the explosive charge is ready, and detonation occurs. The cell infected by the virus is blown open and destroyed, all in a matter of seconds.

The last chemical component making up the defense is *interferon,* a mysterious, nonspecific antiviral substance produced by invaded cells. In what almost appears to be an altruistic gesture by the stricken cell, it produces and excretes interferon not for itself, but for the benefit of neighboring cells that haven't yet come under attack. Although interferon does not act against the virus directly, the chemical appears to strengthen uninfected cells, enabling them to resist invasion of the virus somewhat better than they could otherwise.

Now that we have met all parties to this action, let's take a look at how they interact.

The Struggle

The process begins when a person with active herpes (meaning that sores are present) transmits the virus to someone who is susceptible (not infected), usually during intercourse, in the case of genital herpes, or by kissing, in the case of oral or facial herpes. Since the virus depends on living cells to sustain itself, only this direct skin-to-skin contact allows the virus to enter the cells of a new host.

Having been afforded access to the susceptible cells of a new host, the herpes simplex virus, guided by the most powerful rule of nature—survival—seizes the opportunity and initiates attack. It attaches itself to the outer wall of the target cell and, in a process called fusion, its surrounding envelope becomes integrated with the membrane encasing the cell. When this happens, the virus simply sheds its envelope and finds itself inside the cell.

After gaining entry into the cell, takeover by the virus is swift and relatively straightforward. The virus is transported through the host cell into its nucleus, the center that directs all cellular activity. Here the genetic codes that regulate the normal functioning of the cell are replaced by those of the virus. From this point on, the cell is no longer its own master; all of its energy and raw materials are under the total control of the virus.

With survival hanging in the balance, the rule of the virus is absolute and without mercy. Orders are issued to the cell to terminate its own normal life functions and it is then transformed into a virus factory. For the next twenty hours, the cell will expend its energy and use its resources to produce over twenty thousand exact copies of the herpes simplex virus, each as powerful and determined to survive as the original.

After twenty or so hours of servitude, the infected cell is little more than a shell of its former self. Worn thin and burned out, this hollow remnant of a cell has been damaged beyond repair. All that remains is death.

It will be joined by its neighbors as, one by one, they succumb to the ravaging demands of the virus as it seeks to gain more ground and a better chance for survival. The uninfected cells in the immediate vicinity of their stricken neighbors also come under attack by an expanding army of herpes simplex viruses bent on repeating the cycle of invasion, takeover, replication, and continued cell-to-cell spread. These viruses have no other choice; their complete reliance on cellular machinery for continued existence is as enslaving and driving a force as any they exert over their prey.

When enough cellular death and tissue destruction in a confined area occur, the lesions or sores that are characteristic of active herpes simplex virus disease develop.

The emergence of blisters and ulcers and the appearance of sores are nothing more than the visible markers of the massive battle raging beneath the surface. As the infection worsens, the sores seem to spread over a larger area. If this process of viral invasion, cellular enslavement, and tissue destruction were to continue unabated, in a matter of days blisters and sores would become gaping ulcerations, and in a matter of weeks so much destruction would occur that the victim's life would be threatened. We know this hardly ever happens in cases of herpes affecting persons over three months old—but why not?

The answer is that within the human body the aggressive offensive mounted by the virus in its quest to survive triggers an equally energetic and determined defense to check its internal spread. Far from being a passive victim, the body musters a protective army of specialized cells and chemicals to oppose the invading force.

The Counterstruggle

As we've seen, the object of viral invasion is to seize control of the inner workings of a cell and redirect its functions to produce new viruses. This event is so traumatic that no part of the cell is left unaffected, including the membrane that surrounds it. Almost as soon as the herpes simplex virus invades, chemical changes occur in the makeup of the cell wall that signal the presence of the virus. Macrophages and circulating messenger lymphocytes (B-lymphocytes), which are able to sense the presence of foreign objects in our bodies, detect the cell-wall changes brought about by the HSV and initiate the defense. Macrophages stay and fight while messenger lymphocytes carry word of the invader back to nearby lymph nodes.

Moving in a flowing, amoebalike manner, the fighting macrophages project appendages that surround and eventually encircle the stricken cell containing the virus. When the entire cell has been engulfed by the macrophage, a process similar to food digestion begins: highly destructive acids and enzymes are released to break down the "eaten" cell and dissolve it entirely.

Just as sharks are lured by the scent of blood in water, more and more of these voracious macrophages are chemically attracted from the circulating blood to the site of infection. Each new arrival is greeted by what to it resembles a cellular smorgasbord, and, without the slightest hesitation, it moves in to participate in the feast. The combined predatory action of the macrophages against HSV-invaded cells is enough to slow the infection but not to check it completely, however. Fortunately, the defensive line established by the macrophages receives reinforcement. The dying cells produce interferon, thereby helping still-healthy cells to resist viral attack, and, alerted to the invaders' presence by messenger lymphocytes, B- and T-lymphocytes head straight for the field of action.

Upon arrival, B-cells transform into plasma cells that produce antibodies, which coat the invaded cells. Complement reactions (the binding of C_1 through C_9 on the surface of

infected cells) are initiated, and within minutes the first cellular explosion occurs. As greater amounts of antibodies are
produced by the plasma cells, the explosive pace quickens
and grows in intensity. T-cells contribute to the expanding
defensive action by differentiating into killer cells and lymphoblasts. The killer cells go after cells harboring the virus
directly and attempt to destroy them by releasing lymphotoxin, which is both poisonous and explosive. The lymphoblasts release lymphokines such as maf, mif, and tf, which
serve to amplify and intensify the entire defense.

When all components of the defense are in place and committed to routing the invader, the region of infection resembles a microscopic battlefield: the remains of fallen cells litter
the area, explosions are occurring everywhere, and messengers are being dispatched to bring back a continual stream
of reinforcements. Losses on both sides mount until at some
critical though imprecise point the tide turns and the force
of the defense overshadows that of the challenger.

Invaded cells are being destroyed by the defenders faster
than new cells can be attacked by the viruses, and the cells
that are attacked are eliminated quickly, drastically reducing
the amount of viral replication. As the combined effect of
interferon secretion, macrophage engulfment, antibody formation, complement fixation, lymphokine production, and
lymphotoxin release reaches a peak, viral duplication ceases
entirely and, with each passing moment, fewer and fewer
virus-infected cells are left. Rather than slackening, however, the defense will continue its battle until no cell is left
bearing the surface markers of viral invasion.

In much the same way that the presence of the virus was
sensed originally, so is its absence felt: the lack of virus-
induced cell-wall changes indicate to the body that the battle
has been won and that no further defensive action is needed.
At this point complement reactions are discontinued and B-
and T-cells withdraw and migrate back to lymph nodes. Macrophages remain just long enough to clear the battle scene
of all extraneous matter and battle debris and then withdraw.
The final process, tissue regeneration, begins, and within a
few days healing is complete.

A RECAP

As we have seen, the outward signs of herpes are clues to a furious and complex battle between the virus and the body's immune system. The tingling sensation or itchiness that we feel before sores develop signals the early forward advance of the virus. Cells are being captured and turned into factories manufacturing new viruses, and the growing army of HSV spreads out to invade fresh cells. After a day or two, enough cells have been destroyed so that sores begin to appear on the surface.

As interferon, macrophages, B-cells, T-cells, plasma cells, antibodies, and the complement system begin to take up the defense against the alien force, the cellular field of battle, already crowded, becomes littered with the debris of dead and dying cells. As you might expect, this causes the surface to become swollen and inflamed. The sores may take on a blisterlike appearance as they fill with fluids produced by the defending force. This will continue as long as the defense is still struggling to gain the upper hand; the time varies from person to person.

Once the fluid-filled sores begin to dry and scab over, the turning point has been reached with the defense firmly in control. Swelling, pain, and inflammation begin to subside as T-cells, B-cells, and plasma cells withdraw and macrophages work to clear the area of extraneous matter.

The process of tissue regeneration is initiated as healthy cells duplicate themselves to replace those lost in battle. No longer needed, the scabs fall off to reveal healthy new skin or mucous membrane at the sites of former sores. By this time all surface indications that a battle has occurred are gone, and, with only one difference, our bodies are much the same as they were before exposure to the virus.

The difference is that our immune system will carry the memory of its experience with the herpes simplex virus far into the future. B- and T-lymphocytes will remain sensitive to the specific chemical markers that are unique to HSV. As they make their rounds from lymph nodes through surrounding tissue and back, these patrolling sentries will respond more adeptly and more rapidly should the virus be encountered again. Although the production of antibodies has stopped, whatever amount was produced will continue to circulate in our blood for many months, possibly longer, always on the lookout for the object that originally stimulated their production: an HSV-infected cell.

These lasting changes represent a degree of acquired immunity against herpes. For many people this is enough to ensure no further problems. For others it isn't, although in most cases, because a record of the battle remains, the body's defenses are better equipped to respond to future challenges from the virus. Many people report that the first outbreak of herpes is the worst and that future recurrences are considerably less intense and debilitating.

Our look at the fascinating interaction between the herpes simplex virus and the host is incomplete. The missing dimension has to do with how the viruses manage to survive the devastating counterattack launched by the body and persist in an environment that is lethal to most other microbial challengers.

Earlier we learned that the virus is clever as well as formidable. Confronted by a defense against which further aggression would prove futile, it moves to the relative safety of nearby nerve cells, where, in a state of latency, it escapes detection by its pursuers. But that is only part of the story. For, as we will see in the next chapter, the retreat of the virus into latency is not always the final gesture of a beaten opponent. As stated before, retreat is not necessarily defeat. Although most people don't suffer from repeated attacks of the virus, some unfortunately do; it is the process of recurrences that we will examine next.

CHAPTER 4

———

RECURRENCES: SOMETIMES, ALWAYS, OR NEVER?

———

THE "PROBLEM" DEFINED

Five years have passed since the *Reader's Digest* published Dr. David R. Reuben's article about herpes. Although it was not the first story in the popular press about the disease, it was the most influential in terms of the exposure it received and, in that sense, represented a turning point. Since then, numerous articles have appeared in newspapers and magazines; most of them have been accurate but have tended to focus attention on isolated aspects of the illness, usually the grimmer ones.

Fortunately, recurrent herpes is neither dangerous nor, in most cases, unduly annoying. In terms of numbers, it represents only a small fraction of the total cases estimated to exist at this time. Consider these statistics. Of the 50 to 150 million Americans thought to be harboring HSV-1 or HSV-2, most—roughly two-thirds—don't even know it. They don't get sores periodically and they don't exhibit any outward signs of infection. In fact, the only shred of evidence that indicates they may carry the virus is the presence of the HSV antibodies in their blood as revealed by testing. Since antibodies are specific to microbes, the logical conclusion is that the virus has been or is somewhere in their bodies. Despite its presumed presence, however, recurrence of the virus clearly isn't a problem for these people, and they are in the majority.

Even among the remaining one-third of those harboring the virus, to say that recurrence is a problem is stretching things a bit. Three cases will illustrate the point.

Chuck M. assumes that he contracted labial herpes at age 14, although it's just a guess on his part. All he can be certain of is having first noticed it then. When asked to recall how many times he'd had it since the first time, Chuck, now 33, said, "Maybe twelve times, may be less, but certainly not more." Curious as to where the figure twelve had come from, I asked him how he had arrived at it. "Well," he said, pointing to the sore on his lip, "this is the first one in about three years, and before that I'd get them no more often than once a year, probably closer to once every year and a half. I just divided it out and came up with approximately twelve—though, really, it might be less."

Although eleven years older than Chuck, and certain that she's had herpes since childhood, Claire S. was more definite about her experience. "Once a year, never more, always in the corner of my mouth, and they never last more than five days. It's always the same. We spend every summer on the beach in Sag Harbor. We have a cottage that used to belong to my family, but now Bill and I own it. Almost like clockwork, within the first week of my being there the blisters would form here in the corner, crack open, and within five days would be gone. That would be it. It's the same every year."

Sarah B. tells a slightly different story. She is 26 and became infected with genital herpes in her final year of college. She was perfectly willing to talk about herself. "I didn't know what it was when I first got it," she said. "I don't think the guy who passed it to me did, either. When I went to the Student Health Service, I was frightened. There was a lot of tenderness in the area, and, you know, you think all kinds of crazy things. The doctor who saw me was good. He had an idea of what it was and took some tests to find out for sure. He gave me a cream to lessen the pain and told me to return in four days. When I went back, he said the test was positive and that it was herpes. He didn't do much else medically, but spent a great deal of time telling me about it. I was a lot less worried after that. Even though he said it might come back, he said it probably wouldn't bother me as much. He was right about both. It did come back, several times, but never really hurt again. The only thing I get is a light itch, and in a few days it goes away. I'm not overjoyed about it, but it's not bad at all."

Despite the fact that each of these three persons is classified as having recurrent herpes, none considers it a problem.

In addition to my own clinical observations, there is a mounting body of scientific evidence that clearly reinforces the contention that recurrences have been unduly emphasized and overdramatized.

Noted herpes researcher Dr. Lawrence Corey of the University of Washington School of Medicine has conducted extensive studies to ascertain the differences between primary (first episode) and recurrent genital herpes and reports the following:

> The clinical manifestations of recurrent genital herpes are milder and of shorter duration than initial genital disease. Episodes of recurrent disease are associated with fewer lesions. Recurrent genital herpes has a much shorter duration of symptoms (mean 4.5 days), a shorter duration of viral shedding (mean 4.4 days) [viral shedding is the medical term for how long the active virus persists in lesions], and a shorter time until complete healing of lesions (mean 10.1 days) than that of initial disease. Constitutional symptoms are found only rarely.

In a report entitled "The Natural History of Recurrent Herpes Simplex Labialis," a research team at the University of Utah College of Medicine headed by herpes investigator Dr. Spotswood L. Spruance commented as follows:

Our data confirm and extend previous observations about the short-lived nature of lesions in recurrent herpes simplex labialis. Most lesions progressed from the vesicle [the early point in sore development] to the ulcer/crust stage [the beginning of healing] within 48 hours. Lesion area and pain were maximal in the first 24 hours and declined quickly thereafter. The mean lesion virus titer [the number of viruses present in the lesions] and the frequency of virus-positive lesions were maximal in the first 24 hours and decreased steadily thereafter. *This rapid beginning of natural healing creates a major problem for investigators who seek to hasten resolution further with antiviral compounds.*

And that's the way it is with most of the remaining one-third who periodically experience recurrences. Either because the recurrences are mild or infrequent or because people have adjusted to them, most who get them do not consider them to be a major problem.

This is not to say that recurrent herpes isn't a problem at all. For some people it is, but not nearly as large or sweeping a problem as is often portrayed. As best as I can judge, only a very small proportion of people actually suffer from a chronic and troublesome form of recurrent disease that they themselves would characterize as posing some difficulty.

With this balance in mind, let's then take a look at the phenomenon of recurrent herpes and see how the virus is able to persist despite the best efforts of the body to destroy it.

THE WILL TO SURVIVE

The sequence of events beginning with viral invasion, cell takeover, viral replication, and cell-to-cell spread usually ending with cell destruction is termed *productive infection,* literally meaning that new viruses are produced in the process. The immune response is a direct reaction to productive infection; defense begins as soon as the immune system detects the chemical changes on the surface of invaded cells— almost immediately. The immune response is a potentially devastating one to the virus because the chemical changes it causes in cells will provide constant stimulation for continued defensive activity until every last virus is destroyed.

But nature has endowed the virus with additional powers that enable it to escape annihilation. It can either enter a cell and *not* cause a productive infection or it can enter the network of nerve endings near the site of initial entry and travel along this pathway to nerve clusters called ganglia, where, in a latent form, it can survive indefinitely. Both situations are strategies for viral survival.

In the first situation, HSV invades a cell where one of two things can happen. The first we know of: productive infection. The other result is more defensive than offensive in nature and is termed *nonproductive infection.* The virus enters a cell, but, instead of usurping the cell, the genes of the virus merge with the genes of the cell and there is no detectable disruption. Normal cellular functions are not altered and, as long as the virus remains in this state, no chemical changes on the surface of the cell mark it for destruction by the immune system. It's as though the virus weren't there.

When it comes time for the cell to divide, it does so, duplicating the viral genes along with the rest of the cell. After several reproductive cycles, the original cell may have produced dozens of new cells, each an exact copy of the original "infected" cell and each containing viral genes. Since nothing appears to be wrong, however, no defensive action is taken and the process continues without interruption.

But something *is* wrong. Each new cell contains the complete genetic code of the virus. At any time, one or more of these cells may come under attack—not from without this time, but from within. The viral genes may dominate those of the cell and force the production of new viruses. When this happens, a productive infection occurs, new sores develop on the skin or mucosal surface, and the full cycle of disease is experienced anew. Only this time it is called a recurrent episode.

Many patients wonder whether there can be simultaneous productive and nonproductive infection, and whether an initial contact can result in a wholly nonproductive infection. In the latter case, if symptoms should develop at some time in the future, they would appear to be a primary rather than a recurring episode.

Both cases are possible. The first one—simultaneous productive and nonproductive infection—probably occurs often. The second—nonproductive initial infection—seems to occur but its frequency can't be determined since there is no way to positively distinguish between an initial episode and a recurrence. Interestingly, though, I have seen a number of patients who said they definitely were exposed to herpes but hadn't developed the disease. While it is possible they were mistaken about the exposure, or were lucky and didn't catch the disease, it is also possible that they did, but had a wholly nonproductive infection. I have also seen patients who developed herpes but couldn't explain its origin, since none of the people with whom they had any form of contact had herpes. A wholly nonproductive initial infection some time in the past would certainly explain this puzzle as well.

The other defensive strategy employed by the herpes simplex virus to escape detection and destruction by the immune system is to "hide out" in our nervous system. It seems to have an affinity for nerve tissue.

During the course of a productive infection when new viruses are being manufactured, some, as we've seen, leave the stricken cell to invade neighboring cells and carry the attack forward. Others, however, behave differently; they enter nerve endings at the infected area and migrate along neural pathways to ganglia, nerve clusters far removed from the site of infection.

In the case of labial herpes, these nerve clusters are located near the temples and are called the trigeminal ganglia. In the case of genital herpes, the nerve clusters to which the viruses travel are located alongside the base of the spine and are called the sacral ganglia.

Once the herpes simplex virus has completed its journey and enters the trigeminal or sacral ganglia, it simply remains there in a latent state. Since it doesn't force the production of new viruses by these nerve cells, there is no damage to the nervous system. And, as in the case of a cell housing the virus after it has merged with the cell genes, as long as the dormant virus behaves itself and does not try to take over, the nerve cell shields it by not producing surface chemical markers. The immune system is therefore not provoked and all seems well.

A SYMBIOTIC RELATIONSHIP—SOMETIMES

In Chapter 2, I discussed the relationship between humankind and herpes, pointing out that these viruses were among the most tenacious and successful parasites we have ever known. These characteristics are well illustrated by latency.

For the majority of people who become infected, experience the initial outbreak, recover, and are never bothered again, a perfect union is formed in which the body and the virus coexist in peace and harmony to the detriment of neither. For the entire time that the virus is content to remain dormant, the immune system ignores it and takes no action to disturb the balance. This mating between two normally opposing entities is an example of symbiosis—biologic tolerance between different species or organisms.

Unfortunately, in a small percentage of cases the virus ceases to be content with this arrangement and is reactivated. However, instead of directing its attack against the nerve cells—which is fortunate, because nerve tissue can't be replaced if it is destroyed—the virus retraces the neural pathway it originally took to escape and emerges again at the original site of infection. Here it recovers its aggressive nature and launches a new cellular invasion, and the now-familiar cycle of cell takeover, viral replication, and cell-to-cell spread results in the formation of new sores on the surface of the infected area.

THE SIGNS OF RECURRENCE

Regardless of which mechanism the virus employs to re-emerge, the outward signs are much the same as those of the initial outbreak, with two major exceptions: the early warning signs seem different and the overall experience is less pronounced.

Most people who experience recurrences quickly recognize the often dramatic differences between the first active episode and subsequent ones. To begin with, the *prodrome* —the tingling, itching sensation that precedes the onset of the sores—seems to be more easily detected in recurrences than in first attacks. It's not that the feeling is more intense or worse, but rather that one's ability to sense something going on beneath the surface appears to be sharpened. At least that's what my patients with recurrent herpes report. Most of them can clearly predict a developing outbreak one to two days in advance, and some can feel it three and four days before it happens.

Elena R. gives a good description. "When I first caught herpes, things happened before I really had a chance to note them, particularly the tingles. Now [Elena has had only three recurrences in five years] I can tell days before it erupts, from the pins and needles, only less concentrated. It's like a small part of my lip went to sleep and is just finishing waking up, the very end of the pins-and-needles feeling." Others call it a sense of heat, and some refer to it as a faint itch that is not quite sharp enough to make them want to scratch.

The second notable difference that most patients with recurrent herpes report is far less general physical discomfort. The case of Paul G. is very typical. When I first saw Paul, he had a cluster of approximately eight sores on the shaft of his penis. The area was quite tender and local swelling was pronounced. His inguinal nodes (the lymph nodes of the abdomen) were enlarged and painful, and although he wasn't running a fever, he said he felt "sick" in a general way. This was Paul's initial episode of genital herpes. I told him what I thought it was (later confirmed by lab tests) and how to handle it. I also told him that it might never recur, but that if it did, chances were that it wouldn't hurt as much or make him feel as bad.

I next saw Paul about two years later for a premarital blood test and general checkup. Noting on his record the previous encounter with herpes, I inquired about how he was getting on. "Doctor," he said, "it's almost as you said it would be. For a while, I thought it wouldn't come back at all, but about nine months after the first time it happened again. I would have come to see you, only it wasn't nearly as bad. It didn't hurt much and only lasted a few days instead of nearly two weeks like the first time. And it also happened a few months after that, only then it was even easier. There was hardly any pain and even the sores seemed only halfhearted—they didn't get as bad as they used to."

As I said, Paul's experience with recurrent herpes—less swelling, less pain, less discomfort, even less pronounced development of sores—is fairly typical. Let's examine why this may be so, and at the same time let's look at some of the theories and factors that may influence why some people are subject to recurrences and others, the majority, never are.

IMMUNE STATUS AND RECURRENCES: A DELICATE BALANCE

Today, physicians and researchers engaged in the study of disease and wellness are paying a great deal of attention to the body's natural defense in addition to the agents that cause illness. This is so because, according to the most modern and accurate theories about disease, sickness results not from exposure to an agent alone but from exposure at a time or under a set of conditions when body defenses can't handle the assault. You can see this theory at work constantly. All of us are regularly exposed to cold viruses, influenza viruses, and other microbes commonly found in our environment, yet we are not ill every day of our lives. The agents are roughly the same, but the crucial difference is the power and effectiveness of our natural body defenses at the time of exposure.

Applied to herpes—or to any similar illness that the body must fight unassisted by drugs—differences in the efficiency, power, and effectiveness of the body's natural defenses—collectively termed *immune status*—are probably the most important factors in explaining why some people experience recurrences and others don't. In addition, variations in immune status over time may explain why patterns of recurrence sometimes change as well.

Some of the factors that contribute to immune status are heredity, age, and prior disease experiences, in addition to two factors that are increasingly being regarded as important to herpes—mental attitude (including emotional reaction to life stresses) and behavior. Let's look at each of these.

Heredity, Age, and Exposure: The Basic Factors

The effect of heredity as a factor in immune status is generally considered unalterable. In much the same manner that genetic differences explain why no two people look exactly alike in every external detail, genetic differences explain why no two people are exactly alike in their inherent ability to resist infection and fight disease; their internal detailing is different. Because there is a core of inherited influences on resistance, there are individual differences in the various organs, glands, and other components of each person's immune system; therefore the capacity and function of bone marrow, the lymph system, the thymus gland, and the millions of cells that defend each person are unique to that person and not subject to change.

Age is also a factor that influences immune status and, like heredity, its effect is largely beyond our control. As newborn babies, we lack natural defenses of our own because our immune systems are immature. What little resistance we have has been transferred to us by our mothers, which serves us for the short time it takes our own immune systems to develop. Childhood through middle age is regarded as our period of peak immune status, when we generally resist infection well and bounce back from illness quickly. As we get older, our immune status wanes as we lose some of our former natural capacity to fight off illness. The effect of age on immune status is exemplified by the flu, which is not regarded as particularly dangerous to children, teenagers, and middle-aged adults but can be life-threatening to infants and the elderly.

In addition to heredity and age, prior experiences with disease agents, either naturally through exposure or artificially through vaccination, also influence immune status. It may seem paradoxical, but the more you are exposed to a disease, the greater your immunity to it.

As we have seen, the immune system reacts to a foreign substance only after its presence has been detected in the body. During the first encounter with the substance, detection works in a nonspecific manner. Thereafter, the immune system reacts to specific substances because it retains a memory of the first encounter; this is called the *anamnestic factor.*

As an example of the first case, the various defensive cells such as macrophages and circulating lymphocytes that patrol our bodies are innately able to tell the difference between cells, objects, and substances that do belong in us and those that don't. This ability is nonspecific and is directed against everything interpreted to be "nonself." When a nonself object is encountered, the defense gears up to destroy it, and in the process it becomes sensitized to the unique chemical characteristics of the challenger.

As an example of the second case, if the particular challenger ever turns up in our bodies again, its presence will be instantly and specifically detected. Since the defense is already sensitive to it, less gearing-up time will be required for the immune system to move against it.

This important exposure factor of immune status explains why vaccines afford protection against diseases and why, in the case of most illnesses, once you have had a disease and recovered from it the chances are good that you will never get it again. This factor is also thought to have some bearing on why most people don't suffer recurrences of herpes and why, even among those who do, the recurrences are usually far less troublesome than the first encounter. In a sense, the initial episode is like a vaccine against future recurrences.

Mental Attitude: A Special Factor

Another factor that influences immune status—mental attitude—is a bit more complex than the previous three and requires somewhat more explanation.

The notion that we are more than a complex of proteins, trace elements, and electrochemical energy is about fifty years old. The idea that the mind and body are inseparable and that we can participate in our wellness and/or contribute to our illness—psychically—is now gaining universal recognition and acceptance. There is now enough evidence to support the scientific hypothesis that how and what we think, feel, and believe influence our ability to resist infections and fight disease and that this mind-over-matter influence is very important in herpes.

How? The phenomenon is not entirely understood, but consider the following medical observations that are beyond debate. The adrenal glands located above the kidneys, the hypothalamus region of the brain, and the entire endocrine system, especially the pituitary gland at the base of the brain, respond to emotional stress and anxiety with increased production of several hormones, including adrenalin, cortisone, and pituitary hormone. These hormonal responses are perfectly natural and result in immediate physiologic changes that prepare our bodies to meet the challenge that provoked them. Our heart rate increases, our respiration becomes rapid, our senses become keen, and our energy levels escalate sharply. Our bodies are literally brought to a state of physical readiness to fight or flee. In fact, that is what this complex of physiologic changes is called: the *fight-or-flight response*. It is a primitive and instinctive natural reaction to danger that has proven useful to the survival of all animals, including humans. Nature intended it as an immediate, short-term reaction to be discharged quickly by fighting or fleeing. Once the impending danger has passed, body functions return to normal and, generally speaking, we are none the worse for wear.

Unfortunately, this primitive instinctive reaction is out of place in the twentieth century, for there are few physical dangers that actually require us to fight or flee. Yet we still experience it, not in response to physical threats to our safety but in response to numerous—too numerous—emotional situations and circumstances that upset, distress, worry, or confuse us, situations that really don't allow for an immediate discharge of tension and a rapid return to normal.

When evoked repeatedly or chronically and never quite discharged, the fight-or-flight response can be damaging to one's health. It has been demonstrated that these hormonal changes lower our immune status, making us more susceptible to illnesses if we're exposed to them and less able to control those we already have—like herpes. Since we will be covering this important factor in the next chapter, for now just understand that stress, anxiety, and worry—especially when chronic—are damaging to immune status because they stimulate the fight-or-flight response.

On the other side of the issue, we have all heard or read about the "will to live." This is more than a literary device used by novelists and screenplay writers. Any physician who has cared for a very ill person can tell you that an essential ingredient of treatment is gaining the trust, cooperation, and aggressive support of the patient. It is not known whether this confidence results in a reversal of any damaging hormonal imbalances attributable to prior fight-or-flight reactions or if there are some as yet undiscovered processes triggered by the brain that increase immune status directly, but the positive effect of wanting to be well is profound and recognized by every doctor.

Mental attitude has special importance in herpes. Instead of citing numerous case histories, I feel that detailing the results of recent experiments with ether will demonstrate this to be so. (Since this series of experiments will be covered in depth later, for the sake of brevity some details are omitted here.)

Ether is highly virucidal in a test tube, destroying herpes simplex viruses immediately on contact. This observation led researchers to speculate that applications of ether on herpes sores might speed healing and might even destroy enough viruses to cut down recurrences. The hypothesis was put to the test.

A large number of herpes patients were divided into two groups. One group would receive ether; the other, a substance that resembled ether in every way but was known to have no effect at all on the virus. While the experiment was in progress, neither the investigators nor the patients had any idea which substance was being assigned to which group.

When the experiment was concluded, the codes designating the substances were broken and the investigators began analyzing the data for differences in patient responses. If ether had a beneficial effect, it would show up in the data as a significant disparity between the two groups in pain experienced, lesion severity, the amount of virus present in the sores, healing time, and—possibly—recurrence rate.

The results were disappointing. The data revealed no significant differences in response between patients who had received ether and those who hadn't. On this basis, the hypothesis that ether could be of value in treating herpes had to be rejected.

For the purposes of illustrating the importance of mental attitude in herpes, however, the design and results of the ether experiment are profoundly interesting and valuable even if ether itself didn't prove to be effective.

The design is known as a double-blind placebo-controlled trial, and it is the most acceptable way to test a new drug or therapeutic procedure. All the patients had herpes. All received the same workup, the same tests, and the same care and follow-up throughout. The only difference was that one group of patients received ether and the other group a valueless look-alike substance—a placebo. Until the experiment was over, no one, neither doctor nor patient, knew who had received ether and who had received the placebo (that's what double-blind means).

The major strength of this procedure is its ability to control for a phenomenon known as the placebo effect. Quite simply, the placebo effect is the desire to get well, the hope that a medicine will work, and the wish that the doctor will succeed in curing us. It's all of the positive thoughts, images, and emotions that make up our mental attitude, and it is a powerful factor in every treatment. Since all patients receive some substance and since there is no way to tell the real treatment from the fake, the placebo effect can be controlled.

Wait a minute—this is interesting. By imposing the stringency of placebo-effect control as a part of the most acceptable design for testing new treatments, the medical profession is saying that the placebo effect is an important ingredi- ent of every pill, every injection, and every salve given to a patient. Furthermore, the effect is considered to be poten- tially so strong that not only must it be taken into account, it must also be controlled.

Let's take one last look at the ether experiment to find out how strong is "potentially strong."

As I stated, the outcome of the trial was disappointing. Patients who received ether showed no significant improve- ment over patients who received the placebo—but they weren't worse, either. As a matter of fact, both groups im- proved uniformly. Roughly 75 percent of the group receiv- ing ether reported marked improvement compared to their experience with herpes before treatment, and roughly 75 percent of the group receiving the placebo, known to have no value at all, reported the same kind of improvement. Clearly ether couldn't explain the improvement. Only one thing could: the placebo effect. These patients wanted to improve, and they did.

Even though we've spent a fair amount of time looking at mental attitude as a factor of immune status, the truth is that we've really only scratched the surface. There is so much more to say about handling stress, anxiety, resentment, and guilt, and about building a positive mental outlook and ap- proach in dealing with herpes, that we will cover these im- portant topics in greater depth in Chapter 5. For the time being, however, it's enough that we appreciate the very real physiologic link between our thoughts and emotions and our ability to fight disease, especially a disease such as herpes, which our bodies must fight unassisted by drugs.

Behavior: The Action Factor

The final factor contributing to immune status—behavior— is similar to mental attitude. As is true of mental attitude, the concept that how we behave—how and what we eat, how and when we sleep, how we work, how we play, how we relax, how we dress, and how we spend our energy—has some bearing on our resistance and capacity to overcome illness and is rooted in the same modern view that a human being is more than an aggregate of purely physical parts. Our actions, like our thoughts and emotions, influence the working of those parts.

Obviously, not all behavior counts as an influence on our immune status. Whether we read a book or watch TV between 8:00 and 9:00 P.M. on Thursday makes no difference at all. But what we eat does. So does how we dress when it's cold outside and how much rest and sleep we give ourselves. In general, behavior that affects the functioning of our bodies and our constitutions—to use an old-fashioned word—also influences our ability to fight illness.

The whole issue of behavior as a factor contributing to good health is too broad and sweeping a topic to force into a paragraph or two, and we will be coming back to it in more detail in Chapter 5. For now, the only thing we must recognize is that just as genetics, age, past experience with disease, and mental attitude shape our immune potential, so, too, do some of the behavioral choices we make, particularly in the areas of nutrition, clothing (relative to the environment), relaxation, and sleep.

THE WHY OF RECURRENCE

We have covered much ground in this chapter. We've seen the virus attack for the first time and stimulate a defense against which further aggression is futile. We've seen the virus enter a state of dormancy marked by peaceful coexistence between parasite and host. We've seen the symbiotic harmony of latency shattered as the virus attempts to gain new ground. And we've seen our body defenses, better able to recognize the renewed threat, counter the virus with increased efficiency and effectiveness. We've witnessed a full cycle of action and reaction between offense and defense, with only one element missing—why. What impels the herpes simplex virus to give up the relative safety and security of latency and launch a new attack?

There are two theories to explain the triggering of recurrent episodes. One of them, the nerve-trigger theory, suggests that some form of nervous stimulation causes the latent virus to travel along nerve pathways back to the original site of infection, where it reinvades the skin cells. The other theory, the skin-trigger theory, explains recurrence in a slightly different way.

According to this theory, viral particles are constantly moving from nerve tissue back to skin surfaces in a nearly continuous flow. Most of the time the body's immune defenses are able to eliminate the arriving viruses rapidly and effectively, preventing the recurrence of sores. Sometimes, however, our immune status is not quite up to par, and the virus is able to carry its cellular attack forward and invade enough cells to produce the lesions characteristic of recurrent HSV disease.

Which theory is correct? There is evidence to support and refute both of them, and it's quite possible that elements of both are part of the mechanism of recurrence. Keep this in mind as we further explore mental attitude and behavior in the next chapter.

It may be that some of the attitudinal factors we'll be discussing, such as stress, anxiety, guilt, and anger, not only tend to diminish immune status—in keeping with the skin-trigger theory—but may also provide the nervous stimuli that induce the virus to come out of latency—in keeping with the nerve-trigger theory. It may also be that some of the behavioral factors we'll be discussing, such as nutrition, rest, relaxation, sleep, environmental stress, and trauma of a physical nature, not only lower immune status but result in nervous stimulation as well—in keeping with both theories.

Regardless of what is ultimately discovered to be the exact mechanism leading to recurrence, attitude and behavior are definitely factors, both as influences on immune status and as stimuli of neural activity. An understanding of these variables is crucial to learning to cope with herpes, and the next chapter presents an approach that integrates these and other factors.

CHAPTER 5

WELLNESS AND SELF: COPING WITH HERPES

For the better part of the past several chapters, we've been looking closely at the inner workings of the human body and how it reacts to defend itself against herpes. In this chapter, we will focus on what conscious steps you can take to overcome this disease and achieve wellness.

Recurrent labial and genital herpes can be a painful, miserable, humiliating, frustrating ailment. The sores seem to come and go almost of their own accord. Even though they may produce less physical discomfort during recurrent episodes, the fact that they can't be counted on to stay away is a perennial source of emotional upset for many. The entire experience can be quite tormenting and unsettling for the patient, the patient's family and friends, and the doctor whose care and help is sought.

As frustrating and disquieting as recurrent herpes is to a patient, I can vouch for the fact that it is equally so to a doctor. There are few illnesses that undermine any sense of clinical usefulness and prompt feelings of ineptitude and lack of control to the extent that recurrent herpes does. Patients would develop recurrences and recovery would follow, the entire cycle proceeding quite independently of anything I could do or offer.

Then something happened that changed my thinking about herpes and led to the evolution of a different therapeutic model. Rather than remain committed to a traditional pattern of primary care that had no value for recurrent herpes, I explored a different option that seemed more compatible with what I knew to be the link between the immune system and recurrent herpes. The difficulties some patients experienced were probably the result of individual differences in immune status. If some of the factors influencing immune function could be optimized, patients would have the odds for wellness stacked in their favor.

As a doctor, I had to become more than a crisis-oriented, primary-care body mechanic. I had to become a health educator, a motivator of patient participation in wellness. I had to become a facilitator of health rather than a hands-on repairman, because the tools haven't been developed yet for herpes. By the same token, my recurrent-herpes patients had to adjust as well. They had to learn how to participate in their own wellness. They had to learn how to become activists in a therapeutic process rather than the customary passive objects of a doctor's repair work. And, perhaps most fundamentally, they had to agree to take responsibility for their health.

These positive and comprehensive changes in doctor-patient roles and expectations can also be painful and difficult. Breaking out of long-standing patterns is never easy, and the temptation to regress can at times be powerful. But perseverance pays off in two ways. First, and most important, the approach works. You can make recurrent herpes less of a problem for yourself. Second, the insights you will gain and the changes you will make will serve as a pathway to your general well-being. I have dubbed this pathway the "ABC approach."

THE ABC APPROACH TO COPING
WITH HERPES

A stands for attitude, and in this I include all such thoughts
and emotions as guilt, anger, resentment, anxiety, the desire
to be well, and the commitment to work toward that goal.
B stands for behavior, including attempts to reduce stress,
hygienic techniques to avoid secondary infection, and actions that minimize the risks of inadvertent transfer of the
virus. *C* stands for constitutional factors, such as proper nutrition, adequate sleep, and avoiding unnecessary environmental trauma.

Before we explore each element of the approach, it's important to understand three things: the goal, the interrelat-
edness of all the elements, and the responsibility that you as
patient must accept.

The goal is easy to lay out: learning how to cope with
recurrent herpes. Put another way, it is learning how to
optimize the influences on physical and emotional wellness that we are able to control. Within this context, "success" will be measured in terms of improvement. For
some it may mean less physical discomfort, fewer recurrences, or recurrences of shorter duration. For others it
may mean less emotional distress or less disruption in
their lives. At this time, success does not mean completely
eliminating the virus from our bodies, because this is not
yet scientifically possible. Until it is, learning to cope with
the givens of herpes is our goal.

The second point to understand is that all the key elements
in this overall approach are interrelated. They influence, support, complement, and reinforce each other. There is no
"most important" or "least important" among them. They
are equal and, like the individual notes that make up a chord,
when played in harmony they produce something richer and
more complete than the simple sum of the parts. If one note
is flat or off beat and the whole chord suffers, the would-be
harmony becomes discordance.

The final, and quite possibly the most important, point is
that all the factors in this approach are controlled by one

person alone: you, the patient. For the approach to succeed, you must agree to become an active participant in the process, to translate insights, knowledge, and concepts into dynamic forces for improved health. That is the starting point for this wellness model, as it is for most others.

A: Attitudes for Health

When you agree to accept responsibility for your own wellness, you are taking the first crucial step toward developing a healthy mental attitude. The next steps, however, are not quite as direct, for I have found that many people with recurrent herpes must overcome a variety of negative influences such as anxiety, fear, resentment, and sometimes shame before they can progress further. It is likely that these attitudes are related in part to the misinformation about herpes that is currently circulating—let us call them what they are: myths.

It's extremely rare to find a patient with recurrent herpes who isn't carrying around some negative feelings or mythic beliefs. Most often, during periods of latency, these feelings take the form of anxiety about the next attack and, during periods of recurrence, they may surface as resentment directed against the person who infected him or her, the virus, and the medical profession for not having a cure; self-pity— "why me?"; lowered self-esteem when lip or facial lesions develop; shame (most frequent in cases of genital herpes); fear of spreading it; apprehension that the virus will cause permanent damage.

How do you deal with and ultimately dispose of these negative factors? First, you get rid of the myths. Chapters 1 through 4 have provided you with the facts about herpes and the way the body defends itself against the virus. You now know that the virus is just a parasite and simply wants to survive, that its presence in your body does not constitute a grave danger, that weak natural body defenses may do more to trigger recurrences than any power inherent in the virus. And you know that you can control certain of the factors that influence immune response.

When all this knowledge begins to sink in, you will find your personal view moving closer and closer to the objective reality of the disease. Whatever myths have bogged you down and caused anxiety or fear will suddenly lose their power over you. They will become what they've always been —unreasonable.

Knowing the truth about herpes makes the job of dealing with negative emotions somewhat easier. As a matter of fact, since so much of our negative imagery is often directly related to the virus, the sores, and the unpredictability of recurrences, just gaining greater insight into the physical processes involved can relieve many of our emotional burdens. Some, however, may still remain to be dealt with.

It's been my experience that some recurrent-herpes patients have to work through two additional negative feelings: lowered self-esteem and resentment against the person who infected them. Lowered self-esteem arises in patients with both facial and genital herpes; resentment relates exclusively, or nearly so, to patients with genital herpes. Working out these feelings requires that we understand them, and that we understand how holding these feelings inside diminishes our body's natural capacity to fight the virus.

Lowered Self-Esteem. Self-esteem is the feeling you have about yourself as a *total* human being, the composite image we have of ourselves after factoring in all our doubts and certainties, strengths and weaknesses. Arriving at this image of ourselves is not a static process but a fluid, dynamic one that incorporates and transcends the day-to-day highs and lows. As long as the process remains dynamic, the positives have a chance of canceling out the negatives and we are able to strike a balance in how good we feel about ourselves.

Sometimes, however, the process grinds to a halt. We reach an impasse where some negative gets magnified all out of proportion and the self-corrective dynamic stops functioning. We stop seeing ourselves as the complete people we are and start judging ourselves in terms of the negative.

Recurrent herpes can be the event that creates the impasse and precipitates a lowering of self-esteem. Some patients lose their former sense of attractiveness and feel blemished by the periodic appearance of sores on their lips or faces. Patients with recurrent genital herpes may feel that, somehow, their femininity or masculinity has been compromised. Sometimes they feel as though they are slaves to the virus, a force beyond their control.

Regardless of what shape or form they take, these feelings of diminished self-esteem are irrational, unwarranted, inappropriate, and physically damaging. It is vitally important to correct them—but how? By exploring them, by talking them out with yourself, a friend, a doctor, or, if necessary, a therapist. The case of Christine K. is illustrative of how debilitating lowered self-esteem can be and of how calmly talking through mixed-up feelings can either help you regain a semblance of balance or at least get you to the point of recognizing the need for professional help.

Normally, patients wishing to see me are given an appointment by my receptionist. When Christine called, however, her tone was so frantic and she was so insistent about speaking with me that my receptionist thought it best to summon me to the phone. She was right; Christine's call was not routine. On the line I found a sobbing, somewhat incoherent, and very overwrought young woman pleading that I cure her of herpes because as long as she had it she felt that she had no future. Clearly, she was extremely upset, and I told her to come in immediately.

When Christine arrived she turned out to be a very attractive, well-groomed woman who, on the surface, was the last person you would think had no future. Her initial comments confirmed my first impression; she was intelligent, articulate, and appeared to have everything going for her.

She had contracted genital herpes from Peter, her former boyfriend and one of my patients, whom she had since stopped seeing because she couldn't understand how he could possibly want to be with her any longer. In fact, since contracting the disease, Christine couldn't see beyond it. Her feelings of self-deprecation were summarized by this statement: "Who would ever want me now that I have this?"

We spent a half-hour or so calmly discussing herpes, the facts surrounding her case, and her inappropriate feelings about herself. I pointed out that just as she had accepted Peter as a complete and desirable person even though she knew he had herpes, she too would be perceived as whole and worthy of attention and love despite the disease. I told Christine about the many people I knew personally who continue to date, merit love, give love, marry, and generally live as fulfillingly as before they contracted herpes. I cautioned against allowing this to become a self-fulfilling prophecy: by feeling as she did—however inappropriately—she could begin to behave in ways that would make her undesirable to others, which in turn would reinforce her negative feelings about herself. In fact, Christine admitted that she had already begun to do so: she had accepted and then broken several dates, had rejected the initial advances of several men who wanted to get to know her, and had rebuffed all of Peter's attempts to win her back.

I can't say that our initial conversation, or the two that followed, entirely solved Christine's problem: they didn't. But she did improve. Just talking about her feelings helped lift some of the burden. Most importantly, however, Christine came to realize that she *did* have a problem and sought the assistance of a qualified therapist to help her solve it. I have to believe that she did, for Peter and Christine are now married.

Resentment. Although it occurs far less frequently than loss of self-esteem, another important negative emotion that I encounter is resentment. I hardly ever see it in cases of labial herpes, but among patients with genital herpes it does occur and can be deep-seated. It surfaces in the form of long-term anger and hostility directed against the person (sometimes known, but often unknown) who passed the disease along. It is one of the most confusing, stressful, and physically damaging emotions we can have, for there is rarely an opportunity to release it and we wind up turning it against ourselves. It is essential, therefore, to understand and overcome resentment.

We feel hurt that someone would knowingly or even unknowingly pass this disease to us. But we also feel hostile toward a world in which there is so much ignorance that such a thing could happen. We may also feel helpless about extricating ourselves from the grip of the virus. At the core, though, we can't forgive ourselves for having gotten burned.

Resentment can often be overcome by learning the facts about herpes, by realizing how common an ailment it is and how much is being done to find a solution, and by accepting it as a real physical condition that can be easily managed. Most patients have no trouble seeing that they weren't singled out and that, given its epidemic proportions, there's no one to blame or be angry with. Sometimes, however, a patient exhibits such deep resentment that I can't help but wonder whether herpes merely brought to the surface numerous unresolved hurts and angers that were already there. Barry S.'s case is an example of this.

When I first saw Barry as a patient it was for treatment of a superficial staph infection on his face. He was brooding, sullen, uncommunicative, and obviously worked up about something. I made the diagnosis, prescribed treatment, and told him that he'd be well in no time. He didn't appear to be cheered by this news, so I asked what was upsetting him so much. He said it wasn't the staph infection at all; it was herpes.

It appears that he had contracted genital herpes several years earlier and had been morose and bitter ever since. He was quick to express deep anger at the woman who had infected him and at various doctors he had seen in vain attempts to get cured. He said he had gradually disengaged himself from social ties, and that he neither had friends nor went out on dates.

I pointed out to Barry that for a young man of 27 to have such attitudes and behave in such a way was highly irregular and should be corrected as soon as possible. Barry acknowledged that he didn't much like his present self, but since he had contracted herpes he couldn't help himself. I intimated that he look to more than just herpes for the explanation; of my many patients with the disease, none seemed as disturbed as he. I strongly suggested that he discuss the entire problem with a therapist who could help him understand it better and work it out, for in addition to interfering with his happiness, such deep and chronic resentments would damage his health.

Barry agreed to follow my suggestion and asked for a referral to a psychiatrist. Under the circumstances, just getting Barry to recognize the problem and take constructive action was the best I could hope for. Barry's difficulty—whatever it really was—clearly went beyond herpes and, just as clearly, required the skills of a mental-health professional far more qualified than I.

With or without professional help, if we can get to the point of looking at ourselves, at our own hurt, fears, and feelings of self-admonition ("How could I be so damned stupid?"), we can begin to forgive first ourselves and then others, and get past this damaging thing called resentment.

By not allowing herpes to erode our self-esteem or burden us with resentment and hurt, we do more than improve our psychological state of mind; we improve our physical health as well. Although we've covered this ground before, it is so important that it bears repeating. The mental stresses produced by these negative emotions have a far-reaching effect on our hormonal balance and can ultimately result in diminished immune response. Since we are fully aware that natural body defense mechanisms play a significant role in recurrent herpes, the steps we take to defuse the negative feelings directly influence our health.

From the initial decision to accept personal responsibility for our wellness to the point at which negative feelings cease to burden us emotionally and rob us physically, every step in the process of developing a healthy mental attitude has been conscious and deliberate. This will continue to be true as we build upon those positive attitudes and feelings, rounding out our wellness orientation and the personal forces that will motivate our health-seeking behavior.

B: Behaviors for Wellness

Behavior, the *B* element in the ABC approach, needs no introduction as a factor of wellness. There's hardly a person in the United States who hasn't been exposed to the idea that behavior and health are related. Examples are all around us: smoking and lung cancer, respiratory illness, and cardiovascular disease; oral hygiene and dental cavities; and excessive drinking and liver damage.

As we explore this element of the approach, we will be looking at various forms of wellness behavior that we can adopt for coping with herpes. One of these is the response to stress. Stress is both a detractor from general health and a specific complicating factor in recurrent herpes; this section will raise your consciousness about these aspects and show you the value of destressing yourself. In addition, we will explore special behavior—"tricks of the trade"—that can greatly minimize your risks of secondary infection and eye complications and promote healing. Once you know what you should be doing and why you should be doing it, your preventive efforts will be more meaningful.

Destressing Stress. Stress, more than any other factor, demonstrates the tripartite relationship between our feelings, our behavior, and the functioning of our natural defense mechanisms. Stress is so compellingly linked with lowered resistance to disease and decreased immune system activity that doctors have begun to regard it as having some predictive value in human illness. No wellness approach could be complete without a discussion of this destructive force, particularly one related to herpes. My experience with hundreds of herpes patients has demonstrated that stress is cited more often than anything else as a correlate with repeated and frequent recurrences.

In Chapter 4 we learned about the primitive fight-or-flight response, which is a natural reaction to events we interpret as threatening. We learned that this response results in profound physiologic changes—production of adrenalin, cortisone, and pituitary hormone increases—and, in turn, sharp escalations of pulse rate, respiration, and energy levels. Our senses are heightened and our bodies are primed to fight the perceived threat or flee it, either of which will defuse the response and return our body chemistry to normal. We also learned that modern social conventions stifle the opportunities to physically discharge the response. We are restrained from fighting or fleeing even though we may interpret events as threatening and experience the response. This, then, is stress: the undischarged fight-or-flight response to perceived threats.

The connection between stress and illness was first demonstrated in the 1920s by Dr. Hans Selye at the University of Prague. Dr. Selye's concept of stress holds that any life change or alteration of established patterns can result in the stress response. Events that everyone would agree are negative and threatening—job loss, the death of a loved one, or a near-miss in an automobile—can do this, but so can events that are generally regarded as positive, such as marriage, pregnancy, a job promotion, or a vacation. Dr. Selye uses the terms *distress* to connote stress provoked by negative events and *eustress* to connote stress provoked by positive events. Both kinds of events result in the same stress reaction.

In 1967, Dr. Thomas H. Holmes and Dr. Richard H. Rahe, of the University of Washington School of Medicine in Seattle, conducted an experiment that confirmed Dr. Selye's concepts about stress and its relationship to illness. In their now-famous Social Readjustment Rating Scale, Holmes and Rahe developed a means of assigning numerical values to distressing and eustressing events and surveyed several thousand people in order to measure the amount of stress in their lives.

On the basis of the scores achieved, the investigators were able to predict illness with a high degree of statistical accuracy. Those whose lives were stressful had 90 percent more illness than those whose lives were not.

Stress brings about a diminution in immune response because antibody formation, lymphocyte function, and macrophage activity are hampered by hormonal surges. At the University of New South Wales in Australia, Dr. R. W. Bathrop demonstrated the effects of depressed B- and T-lymphocyte function in people experiencing the stress of bereavement. Since B-cells become antibody-producing plasma cells and T-cells become lymphoblasts and killer cells, every aspect of the immune system suffers when these cells are affected.

The implications of stress-induced immune system depression for people who have herpes are clear: since the control of recurrences depends on immune status, any factor that lowers it can cause more difficulty. In addition to lowering immunity, the nervous agitation that accompanies stress may stimulate viruses to leave nerve tissue where they have been lying dormant. Controlling stress, therefore, is fundamentally important.

Much has been written about stress reduction and, rather than repeat all the methods, techniques, and exercises that have been proposed for reducing stress, I have provided several suggestions for additional reading on the subject in the reference section at the back of this book.

As a preface to any additional reading you may do, I offer the following observations:

Any alteration in your life—big, small, positive, or negative—can cause stress; the essence of stress is change.

Many stresses in life can be controlled by anticipating the events that provoke them and either removing them, changing them, or spacing them out over time. By limiting anticipated stress, unanticipated stress that occasionally occurs may be less damaging.

Learning to relax, think clearly, and remain calm during unexpected stressful events will help defuse them and diminish their damaging potential.

The effect of stress can be cumulative. Chronic stress is the most damaging; clusters of stressful events in a short period of time are somewhat less damaging.

In conclusion, how you behave in relation to stress—the extent to which you are able to anticipate and avoid it and the techniques you employ in coping with the stress you can't avoid—has great bearing on your immune status and the ability of your natural defenses to hold the herpes virus in check. Anything you do to reduce the negative effects of stress on your immune system will improve your chances for achieving wellness.

Sidestepping Secondary Infections. Since the lesions caused by the herpes simplex virus are breaks in skin or mucosal surfaces, our approach to wellness must include an understanding of what these breaks mean, what dangers they may create, and how to avoid them.

Nature has provided us with an outer covering of skin and mucous membranes as the first line of defense against most of the microorganisms with which our bodies come into contact. When this external barrier is unbroken, germs have little opportunity to gain entry and infect us. However, when the skin is abraded, cut, or torn and the integrity of the barrier is compromised, microbes can enter freely. Under normal conditions, when exterior tissues and those lying just beneath the surface are healthy, natural body defenses are usually enough to counter any foreign organisms that get in.

For people with recurrent herpes, however, the situation may be somewhat more difficult. The ulcerated sores of herpes, like cuts or wounds, provide portals of entry for infecting bacteria. But, unlike simple cuts or wounds, these openings are the result of a process in which tissues at the surface and just beneath have been diseased, traumatized, and destroyed by the virus. Because such tissues are already in a weakened state, any bacteria that find their way in may face less resistance than otherwise might be the case. The secondary infection that might result could be stubborn, painful, distressing, and sometimes dangerous. To avoid such a condition, we have to give nature a helping hand.

Contrary to popular belief and frequent practice, antibacterial and corticosteroid creams such as Neosporin, Mycolog, and Valisone; antiseptic preparations such as Bactine, First Aid Cream, Blistex, and Camphophenique; and even lemon juice are *not* recommended or desirable. According to Dr. Lawrence Corey, a prominent herpes-simplex-virus expert at the University of Washington School of Medicine, such creams and ointments tend to spread the virus around, increase new lesion development, and generally delay healing.

The practice most widely recommended by herpes virologists and clinicians to minimize the risk of bacterial secondary infection and promote healing of the sores is to keep them dry and clean. Cleansing with water (and soap, if it is not painful) is sufficiently hygienic. The use of drying agents such as epsom salts or Burrows solution applied locally and then allowed to air dry is also acceptable. And, obviously, the less you touch the sores with your fingers, the less chance there is of introducing unwanted bacteria.

If despite your hygienic precautions you still develop a bacterial infection at the site of the lesions, go to your doctor at once for prompt diagnosis and proper treatment.

Avoiding Autoinoculation. Autoinoculation, the self-transfer of the virus from one part of your body to another, usually by touching, is an important subject to learn about and an important complication to guard against.

If left alone, herpes sores rarely crop up at a site other than where the virus initially entered the body, and recurrences of both labial and genital herpes will usually produce lesions within millimeters of the original infection. Unfortunately, we don't always leave the sores alone, and at times we aren't even aware that we've touched them. In these situations the spread of the virus is quite possible. For example:

The sores sometimes itch; you scratch them.

You feel the first tingle of a sore coming up; you constantly probe the area to monitor its progress.

You have genital lesions and can't avoid touching them when you urinate.

While smoking a cigarette, you inadvertently touch the sore on your lip.

While writing or thinking, you unconsciously rest your chin in the palm of your hand and your fingers brush against your lip sores.

You wear contact lenses and use saliva as a wetting agent, not even thinking of the sore on your lips.

When you wake in the morning, not realizing that you may have scratched your sores in your sleep, your first act is to rub your eyes.

I could go on with this list, and it would probably cover the better part of two pages, but I don't think it is necessary. My point is simply this: these unconscious acts can easily transfer the virus to a new location, resulting in recurrences at one or more new sites. Worse, however, is the possibility of introducing the virus into your eyes, which can result in partial or complete vision impairment.

These complications of herpes can be totally avoided if you take certain preventive measures. First, when sores are present, make a conscious effort not to touch, scratch, pick, or otherwise explore the lesions. This may be difficult at times, but it's the best way to avoid spreading the virus to a new location, including your fingers, which are vulnerable, too, especially if you have a cut or other opening in the skin. Try to be aware of what you do with your hands.

Second, if you realize that you have accidentally or inadvertently touched the infected area, immediately wash your hands with soap and water.

Third, incorporate the following behavioral rules into your wellness consciousness.

Always wash your hands thoroughly with soap and water during a recurrence. Make this your first act when you get up in the morning (before you rub your eyes) and repeat it each time you touch the sores.

Never use saliva as wetting agent for contact lenses if you have labial herpes, even when you *aren't* experiencing a recurrence.

Never insert contact lenses without having first washed your hands with soap and water, no matter where your herpes infection is located.

If you follow these simple rules, the chances of transferring the virus to new locations will be minimized.

If, despite your best attempts to guard against self-transfer of the virus, you develop an eye infection (it feels like you have something in your eye and it looks like a bad case of conjunctivitis, or "pink-eye"), don't despair. Go to your doctor immediately. If it's herpes keratitis, it can be treated effectively, and the sooner the better.

C: Constitutional Factors for Wellness

As we explore this final element in the ABC approach, we will be looking at three general influences on your constitutional well-being: nutrition, sleep, and the external environment. All three influences are important to health in general, particularly if you happen to have herpes. If you keep your body in the best possible condition it will help you achieve and maintain your immune potential—the vital factor in controlling recurrences.

Nutrition. Your body is made up of between 60 and 100 trillion cells, each cell a unit of life unto itself, the fundamental component of living things. Cells have various shapes, sizes, and functions. For example, nerve cells transmit impulses and red blood cells carry oxygen. Others work together to form our various internal and external structures, and still others—the 100 billion-plus army of macrophages, lymphoblasts, plasma cells, and killer cells—are the vital components of our natural defense against disease.

Regardless of their specific duties, each of these trillions of cells is like a miniature industrial complex, manufacturing its own energy, keeping its machinery in good working order, effecting repairs when necessary, maintaining close surveillance over what comes in and what goes out, and, from time to time, building a new plant (nerve cells are the major exception to this last point; they don't reproduce). And, again like industrial complexes, cells require fuel supplies and raw materials to maintain operations and function effectively.

It is important to provide the body's cells with the fuel they need to keep running at peak efficiency and the raw materials they need to make repairs and build new components. This is the principal biologic objective of eating for physical well-being, and we can achieve this essential goal when we bring our eating behavior into line with our wellness orientation. In order to have a healthful diet that is balanced and adequate, we must become aware of the nutrients our cells need to function properly and, if necessary, alter our eating habits to fulfill these needs.

The following overview of the necessary elements of a balanced diet is meant to serve as a guide against which you should examine your own eating behavior and the extent to which it is in harmony with your orientation to be well. There's no pat answer in terms of what constitutes good eating habits. Clearly, there are many variations of diet that can provide nutritional sufficiency. By the same token, individual nutritional needs differ depending on a variety of factors, including how much alcohol we consume, how much we smoke, how much physical exercise we get, how old we are, and whether we are male or female.

Think about eating and nutrition as behavior that you can control. Try to spot deficiencies and, more important, try to correct them. If you are in doubt about the adequacy of your diet, talk to your doctor about it or read any of the books suggested in the reference list. You owe it to yourself because you deserve to be well. And remember, just as mental attitude, hereditary factors, and age affect the performance of your 100-billion-cell immune defense army, so does the quality and sufficiency of the nutrients you provide to these vital protectors of your health.

Carbohydrates. Carbohydrates are a class of essential nutrients that serve as the primary and most immediately available source of fuel for your cells. In addition, carbohydrates assist in regulating protein metabolism and in breaking down fats by the liver. In food, carbohydrates primarily take the form of starches, sugars, and cellulose. Of these, starches are among the best sources of carbohydrates because they are easily digested and converted to glucose—a simple sugar that is the body's most efficient fuel source—which is carried by the blood to every cell.

Foods containing adequate supplies of starches are grains, legumes, and vegetables, all vital components of a balanced diet.

Fats. Fats constitute another class of essential nutrients that serve as a source of fuel for your cells; however, they are secondary to carbohydrates and are not immediately available for use. Fats are not water-soluble and therefore must be broken down by liver-bile acids before they can enter the system for use by cells. Fats also serve as raw materials for such structures as the cell membrane.

Food substances containing saturated fats are meat, butter, milk and milk products, and eggs (primarily the yolk). Foods containing unsaturated fats are vegetables, vegetable oils, margarine, and nuts. Saturated fats contain cholesterol whereas unsaturated fats do not. Since elevated cholesterol levels cause problems for some people and since cholesterol is produced by the body naturally, you may wish to consult your physician about which sources of fats would be best for you.

Proteins. Protein is one of the most essential nutrients for cellular maintenance and growth, as it is the major source of raw materials for the cells that make up muscle tissue (including the heart), blood, skin, many vital organs, and nerve tissue. Proteins are actually complex molecules formulated by smaller parts called amino acids. The human body is able to produce all the amino acids it needs except for the following eight: isoleucine, leucine, lysine, methionine, phenylalanine, threonine, tryptophane, and valine. These are known as essential amino acids because they must be furnished in our diets.

Foods containing all eight essential amino acids are called complete protein foods and include most meats and dairy products. Foods containing fewer essential amino acids are called incomplete protein foods and include most fruits and vegetables. Certain combinations of incomplete protein foods, however, will provide all eight essential amino acids. Regardless of what source of dietary protein you choose, you must provide your body with an ongoing supply if your cells are going to operate at the optimum level.

Vitamins. Vitamins are a class of organic compounds that are necessary for the normal uptake and use of other nutrients by cells. They act as catalysts to facilitate chemical reactions that cause nutrients to be used for producing energy and for building and maintaining cells and tissues. With few exceptions, vitamins cannot be manufactured by the body and, like the eight essential amino acids, they must be supplied in the diet or through supplements. Most vitamins are water-soluble, which means they are readily available for use by cells. It also means that they cannot be stored in the body; excess quantities are eliminated in urine. Therefore, the body's supply of water-soluble vitamins, mainly vitamin C and the B-complex, must be replenished on a regular basis, usually daily. In contrast to vitamin C and the B-complex, vitamins A, D, and E are fat-soluble and *can* be stored by the body, to be moved out of reserve and used as needed. To prevent depletion of these reserves, it is important that they be replenished frequently.

Today, as in the past, diet alone can provide all the vitamins you need. As a result of improper food preparation, overprocessing, or restricted food intake for weight control, however, the vitamin content in food may not be sufficient and supplements may be necessary. It's best to consult your physician before choosing a vitamin supplement.

Minerals. Minerals are inorganic compounds that make up 4 to 5 percent of an average person's body weight. Their role in cellular health is essential despite the relatively small amounts usually present. Iron, for example, is needed by blood cells to carry oxygen throughout the body and take away carbon dioxide. Calcium is necessary for the health and well-being of such hard tissues as bones and teeth and of the membrane surrounding every cell. Zinc is particularly important to the cells that make up skin. In combination with other nutrients and compounds, minerals affect almost every vital body function.

As with most vitamins and the eight essential amino acids, minerals are not manufactured by the body and must be supplied through food or mineral supplements. The mineral content in a balanced diet is generally sufficient for most people, but dieters or persons who tend to concentrate on certain foods may not be getting a proper mineral balance. In this case it is well to consult with a doctor about the need for mineral supplements.

The foregoing overview of nutrition illustrates the need to carefully consider proper foods as the cornerstone for a healthy constitution, a necessity for attaining wellness.

In Chapter 10 we'll examine in more detail the claims that two nutritional elements—vitamin C and zinc—may play an important role in coping with herpes.

Sleep. As everyone knows, sleep is a physiologic need. We cannot survive without it. During sleep, our minds and bodies undergo a form of rejuvenation. Energy that during waking hours is spent on moving, thinking, and interacting with the external world is turned inward during sleep. Repairs are effected, the machinery of our bodies is recharged, and our minds get a needed break as well. The tensions and anxieties of our waking lives are given a chance to work themselves out while we sleep. In every sense, sleep tunes our bodies and minds, helping to keep us in peak condition so that we can face the physical and mental demands of conscious activity.

Obtaining adequate sleep is very important for people who have herpes. Too little sleep deprives your body of the time it needs for physical reconditioning and has a negative impact on your mental attitude, leaving you irritable, anxious, and poorly prepared to handle the many taxing situations that arise every day. And, as we already know, a positive mental attitude is one of the key elements of wellness.

When you chronically get too little sleep and become run down, every part of your body is affected. The resulting physical and mental fatigue can detract from your general stamina and feeling of well-being and hamper the performance of your immune system.

How much sleep is enough? Since sleep requirements are highly individual, there is no set rule for everyone, although few people can get by with fewer than six hours a night and most need between seven and nine hours. Your best guidepost is how you feel upon awakening. If you wake tired and drowsy and have difficulty becoming mentally alert, you are probably not getting enough sleep and should try to get more. The last thing you want to do is realize that you haven't been getting enough sleep by experiencing fatigue and exhaustion.

The External Environment. In addition to such internal factors as mental attitude, the effect of stress, and nutrition habits, our general health and, in particular, our immune status, is affected by external environmental factors, including extremes in weather. And some external factors, such as intense sunlight, wind, extreme dryness, and physical irritations that traumatize the site of infection, may directly aggravate recurrent herpes.

The idea that physical environment may be a factor in lowering resistance, promoting disease, or complicating existing conditions is not new. In fact, it's one of the first disease-related concepts we learn at an early age. Who can forget our parents' endless admonitions to wear a sweater so we won't catch cold? And anyone who lives in a city has heard the terms *smog-alert* and *air-quality index,* and warnings to people with chronic respiratory conditions to remain indoors.

Exposure to adverse environmental influences is of special concern in recurrent-herpes patients as well, for if we fail to take the proper precautions against environmental abuses, we may exacerbate an otherwise stable situation.

Let's start with that parental charge to dress warmly to avoid catching a cold. Cold weather doesn't cause colds; viruses do. But being cold can diminish your immune capacity and put you in a state of lowered resistance, making you more vulnerable to cold viruses. This applies to herpes because, as we know, recurrences may result from the stifling of immune response. Since the goal is wellness and dressing inadequately for cold weather can lower resistance, you should dress appropriately for the weather. This may seem like a trite statement of the obvious, but in this fashion-conscious world you'd be surprised how many motivations other than health influence what we wear.

Both cold and hot weather require precautions on the part of those with recurrent labial herpes. If you are one of these people, avoid getting chapped lips, because lips that are cracked and peeled have been "environmentally traumatized." Such abuse leaves them in a weakened state and may make a recurrence more likely. Use a lip salve to keep your lips from drying out and avoid licking or rubbing them.

Also of some concern to those with labial herpes is the effect on the lips of direct sunlight, particularly the concentrated rays found on ski slopes and at beaches. Exposure to intense sunlight is abusive, damaging, and dangerous in any case, but for someone with labial herpes it is especially so. The ultraviolet radiation can cause local tissue destruction; it is extremely common for recurrent-herpes patients to suffer reactivation of the virus after exposure to intense sunlight. If possible, avoid such exposure entirely; if you must be in the sun, take it in moderation and coat your lips with an effective sun-screening agent.

This same advice applies to climates where there is constant wind or extreme dryness, both of which can dry out and chap your lips. The use of a lip salve is recommended to prevent this.

Most of these direct traumatic environmental influences don't affect people with recurrent genital herpes because the genitals are so well protected, but there is one that does: sexual intercourse. Many patients report recurrences of the virus following prolonged or unusually vigorous sexual activity. Considering the friction involved, it makes some sense that prolonged or vigorous intercourse may serve to abrade vaginal tissue or the skin surface of the penis. The solution may be to ensure adequate lubrication, either naturally or with lubricating jelly.

For both the labial and genital herpes patient, behavior that promotes constitutional well-being and minimizes environmental trauma makes sense. Sometimes the choice of behavior requires some preliminary detective work in order to find patterns in your recurrences and relate them to some factor in your environment. Let me give you three examples from my practice to illustrate what I mean.

Andy, who has oral herpes, deduced that a pattern of several recurrences in rapid succession might have been attributed to eating pizza that hadn't cooled sufficiently. According to him, the sores reappeared after he had burned his mouth on hot pizza. He is convinced that his deduction was correct, because he now allows the pizza to cool before putting it in his mouth and doesn't experience recurrences as frequently as he had.

Cynthia, who has labial herpes, surmised that her habit of scraping her top teeth across her lower lip might be implicated in her recurrences. She asked me about such a possibility and I said it was plausible; the constant scraping might injure her lower lip and make a recurrence more likely. I suggested that she consciously stop doing it and see what happened. After several months she seemed convinced that the scraping had been at least a partial factor; after she stopped doing it, her recurrences were less frequent.

Lorraine believed that the chafing from her tight-fitting synthetic underwear might be aggravating her case of genital herpes, and reported that after switching to cotton underwear her recurrences were less frequent.

ALL FACTORS CONSIDERED

I'd like to conclude this chapter with a composite observation based on patient experiences with this wellness model. If you have the conviction to adopt the ABC approach, and if you have the determination to stay with it, I guarantee that you will achieve personal mastery over recurrent herpes in any or all of the following ways.

1. To the extent that recurrent herpes has been a major encumbrance in your life, you will find it to be far less so.

Recurrences will cease to cause you major emotional disruption and will become minor inconveniences of little consequence.

2. You will experience less physical discomfort when you do suffer a recurrence—partly because you are giving your body's natural defense mechanisms all the support you can, and partly because your perceptions have changed.

3. You may experience fewer outbreaks or find that sores heal more quickly.

4. You will be healthier and happier knowing that, to the fullest possible extent, you are a force in your own wellness.

5. You will be better able to accept your responsibility for prevention and more likely to be successful at accomplishing it. For, as we will see in the next chapter, with an infectious epidemic such as herpes, wellness and self is only part of the story.

CHAPTER 6

WELLNESS
AND OTHERS:
PREVENTION

Disease prevention is an idea whose time has come, not just in terms of herpes, but in relation to all illnesses that affect humans. We can see indications of this all around us.

Just ten years ago, the concept of a Health Maintenance Organization (HMO)—a group medical practice structured to provide services to maintain the health of its members rather than to respond to crises (illness) as do traditional primary-care models—was the futuristic dream of a few visionary health planners and public-health officials. Today, with modest government subsidies to pilot the concept and develop it, the HMO is a reality with several in full operation throughout the country.

Just ten years ago, health insurance was really sickness insurance, with premiums paid in anticipation of illness and benefits returned only on the basis of a diagnosed medical problem. Today, health-insurance benefits cover a broad range of prevention services, such as the PAP test, special nutritional counseling, vaccinations, and periodic checkups. In addition, some insurance companies are experimenting with new plans that are truly prevention- and wellness-

oriented. Premiums paid would cover preventive-health services and indemnify against catastrophic loss in the event of
serious illness, but if the insured person remained healthy
and didn't use the latter benefit, a portion of the premiums
paid would be returned—a reward for keeping healthy.

Just five years ago, prevention was a word rarely heard at
medical seminars and meetings. In just the last three years,
the Department of Health, Education, and Welfare sponsored a massive nationwide study that not only dealt with
prevention but was actually called the Task Force on Prevention. I had the honor of participating in that study and can
tell you firsthand that the focus was not on illness but on what
the doctors and allied health professionals of this nation can
do to promote wellness. The enthusiasm and interest expressed by the thousands who participated stimulated the
most aggressive governmental prevention effort ever under-
taken: the establishment of wellness targets to be achieved
by the year 1990, with plans and strategies to be employed
to accomplish them.

From my own practice I could cite numerous examples of
the growing interest in prevention, but if forced to choose
one that I consider most telling, it would have to be this: Just
a short time ago there was a natural temptation on the part
of parents, teachers, and school nurses to question a student's
illness. Was it real or just a ploy to stay at home? Often I could
detect a dual motive when parents wanted me to examine
their children: concern about their child's health along with
a need to verify that something was indeed wrong. The pro-
verbial "note from the doctor" requested by schools after an
absence of several days reflected the same need to make sure
that the child was really ill.

Now parents tend to call me not because they suspect
faking but to make sure their child can return to school
without the risk of infecting classmates. And the same sort of
prevention attitude is evident among school officials. School
nurses frequently call to verify that a child's cold, flu, or other
illness is no longer communicable. Quite a change, I'd say,
and one for the better.

THE NECESSITY OF PREVENTION

Why all this interest in prevention? Is it just the current trend that will pass with time? While prevention certainly is in vogue, it's more than that: prevention is a necessity.

There are two main reasons for this concern with prevention. The first is the rapidly rising cost of crisis-oriented medical care; the second is that crisis medicine just doesn't work in some situations.

The fact that hospital charges, physician fees, and laboratory costs have more than tripled in the past ten years concerns everyone. In purely economic terms, the financial burden of illness is killing us, and it's a burden borne by everyone in the form of higher taxes, higher insurance premiums, and higher out-of-pocket medical costs. The writing on the wall is clear for all to see: this country can no longer afford the luxury of getting sick. The state-of-the-art, high-technology, crisis-care system we elaborately constructed over the past twenty years is simply too expensive to maintain. While it can't be shut down, it can be trimmed selectively and reserved for only those situations that demand it. Preventing illness is the key to accomplishing this financially mandated goal.

In addition to the economic lesson we are being forced to learn, medicine is rapidly awakening to another harsh but important reality: for all our modern gadgets, computer-assisted devices, and high-technology equipment, the prognosis for certain illnesses that are brought to our attention as after-the-fact crisis conditions is not much better today than it was twenty years ago. The overworked, overweight, underexercised patient who suffers a massive heart attack is a little better off today, but not much. We can do a bypass if it's indicated and we can monitor every minute detail of heart function with a precision undreamed-of in the past, but if the damage is great, there's really not much we can do.

The heavy smoker whose lungs become cancerous or who develops emphysema is in a sad state even today. So is the chronic hypertensive who suffers a stroke or kidney damage. These are all conditions for which there is very little effective therapy, even if only one lung becomes cancerous or only one kidney stops working. Once a disease reaches the crisis stage, there's little that can be done.

Preventing these and many other illnesses, therefore, has become a central concern of cardiologists, thoracic surgeons, radiologists, neurologists, cardiovascular specialists, and others. Of course, treatment is still a major theme, but it has been outpaced by a more important one—prevention.

In addition to these obvious motivations for a greater focus on prevention, there is one other: responsibility. Whether it is an outgrowth of holistic medicine, the wellness movement, the human-potential movement, or just a natural consequence of humanity's evolution, the idea of free choice, with its corollary of taking responsibility for our choices and actions, is taking hold and leading to the widespread practice of prevention.

Today, more than at any time in the past, people are concerned about their health and choosing responsible pathways to preserve it. This can be seen in our decisions not to smoke (or at least to smoke a low-tar brand), to eat more healthful foods (and how we prepare them), to be more aware of our bodies and quickly respond to signs of illness, and to do countless other life-affirming things to express a protective reverence for continued good health.

This notion of responsibility and prevention naturally extends beyond ourselves. We know we don't live in a vacuum. We know that the actions of others—food producers using pesticides, industries dumping wastes into our water supply and spewing forth toxic matter into the air we breathe, inconsiderate people letting loose with uncovered coughs and sneezes in our midst—affect the health we responsibly try to preserve. And we resent these things when they threaten us.

But the extension of responsibility and prevention beyond ourselves runs two ways. Just as we expect others not to threaten our health, we must make sure that our actions don't create health hazards for others. As we are about to see, this latter point has special importance in herpes.

THE RESERVOIR CONCEPT

Public-health officials and epidemiologists (doctors specializing in epidemics) frequently consider communicable diseases such as herpes as analogous to a series of reservoirs at various levels of fullness. One is the *reservoir of susceptibles,* symbolically containing all people at risk of catching the illness; another is the *reservoir of infectiousness,* containing all infected people who can spread the disease; a third is the *reservoir of infected,* containing those people who have the illness in a noninfectious form and who can therefore neither give nor get it; and, finally, the *reservoir of nonsusceptibles,* containing people who have been vaccinated for immunizable diseases or who for any other reason can't get the disease.

As applied to most infectious diseases for which vaccines or cures exist or which are infectious only for a short time, the reservoir concept is a dynamic model with constant movement between reservoirs. Susceptibles are vaccinated and become nonsusceptible. Infectious people cease to be so over time and are merely infected. Infected people get better or receive treatment and become either nonsusceptible or susceptible, depending on whether or not the disease confers natural immunity (for example, the mumps does; a staph infection does not).

Viewed in this context, epidemic control has three simultaneous objectives: (1) to identify, treat, and immunize (sometimes the disease itself is the immunizing agent) as many infectious people as possible; (2) to make as many susceptible people as possible nonsusceptible by vaccine or isolation; and (3) to find and treat those who are infected but not infectious, even though they don't threaten anyone.

Obviously, this model works best when applied to diseases that are curable and immunizable (either naturally or artificially), but it also works well if it is only curable. Syphilis is an example of a nonimmunizable disease that was brought under control simply by curing enough people. Even though cases still occur, the reservoir of infectiousness is so low that it no longer represents an epidemic threat.

Unfortunately, the model doesn't work at all when applied

to a disease that is neither immunizable nor curable, such as herpes. In this case, the flow between reservoirs is not dynamic at all: it's all one way. Since nearly everyone who doesn't already have herpes is susceptible, exposure results in either the enlargement of the reservoir of infectiousness or the enlargement of the reservoir of infected. Without a cure to inhibit this process, these reservoirs keep getting larger as new susceptibles are exposed and infected. And there is an additional problem. As the size of infected and infectious reservoirs grow, the rate at which new susceptibles catch herpes increases, since the opportunity for exposure is constantly expanding.

Unless we deliberately intervene in this seemingly interminable process, the reservoirs containing people with herpes will increase geometrically (1, 2, 4, 8, 16, 32, and so on), and eventually nearly everyone will have herpes.

Frightening? Yes. Hopeless? Not at all. Even though we presently lack both a cure and a vaccine, we can still employ a nonmedical-intervention strategy to curb the epidemic— in a word, prevention. Fortunately, as we are about to learn, in addition to its strengths, herpes has some weaknesses, and by exploiting the natural weaknesses of herpes, prevention is not only possible, it's easy.

HERPES: AN INFECTIOUS DISEASE FOR ALL SEASONS

Herpes owes its prolonged existence as a human illness to several important factors. These viruses are able to persist in a host indefinitely, they are able to recur from time to time, and they are highly infectious. Had nature failed to endow them with any one of these powers, it is doubtful that the disease could have flourished.

If infection led to severe illness and death, these viruses would perish with the host and most of us would be spared. Pockets of disease would spring up here and there, and in a relatively short time all those who contracted herpes would die; thus the epidemic would literally burn itself out.

If the disease never recurred, only the initial episode would be infectious, and the opportunities for transmission would be sharply curtailed. Not only would the number of people infected be far smaller than it is today, but the facility with which the viruses span generations would be greatly reduced.

And, obviously, if these viruses were even slightly less infectious, transmission would be a much smaller concern, as would the extent to which the disease is entrenched in the population.

Unfortunately, nature has superbly equipped the herpes simplex virus for survival. But, interestingly, as important as these natural endowments are, had it not been for the unwitting cooperation of humankind itself, herpes would not be nearly the problem it is today and, in fact, might not exist at all.

It is easy to understand why. Primarily as a result of imperfect knowledge (the germ theory of disease is relatively new), there has been little or no emphasis placed on curbing the spread of this disease. Because people didn't know better, they provided the herpesvirus with the one thing nature had left to chance: constant exposure and access to new hosts.

But today we know better. While our understanding of herpes is still imperfect, it is more complete than ever before and is certainly sufficient to allow us to exploit the major natural weakness of these viruses—the manner in which they are transmitted—and successfully accomplish what should have been done before: prevention.

Extending the wellness model to others by practicing prevention presupposes that you understand how and when herpes can be transmitted and that you learn what to do to reduce the possibility of its spread. Let's explore each of these important aspects separately.

The Facts About Transmission

Herpes is known as a human-contact disease. The infectious agent, the virus, is transmitted from person to person by direct contact. While it is theoretically possible for the virus to be spread by inanimate objects, such as an unsterilized surgical instrument or a drinking glass shared with a person who has labial sores, these methods of transmission are both unlikely and highly remote. Nearly 100 percent of all cases of herpes are spread directly from one person to another.

When I explain this fact to my patients, some of them start to get nervous and fidgety. The mention of a direct-contact disease makes them think of those other well-known contact diseases, the ones nice people aren't supposed to get. Occasionally a brave soul will come right out and ask, "You mean herpes is something like those social diseases?" To which I usually reply, "Sure, herpes is a lot like pink-eye and staph infections, and be thankful for it. It's even like VD sometimes."

There is absolutely no reason to be distressed about the notion of contact transmission. It's purely descriptive, without any ethical, religious, or moral overtones. People don't react to the other media in which diseases are spread—air, water, insects, animals—and they shouldn't react to this one, either. As a matter of fact, because herpes can be spread only by direct contact, prevention is a real possibility. If the disease were transmitted in the air, prevention would be more difficult or even impossible, much as it is with the common cold.

Direct contact, therefore, is mandatory for the infection to be passed along. And by direct contact, I mean anything from as simple and common a human gesture as a kiss to as tender and meaningful an act as sexual intercourse. When conditions are right, these very natural, everyday activities can result in the transmission of herpes.

Fortunately, conditions are not always right. This, then, is a second factor that makes prevention a real possibility. Direct contact such as kissing or sex are significant only when viruses are present on skin or mucous-membrane surfaces. And, as we have seen already, this happens only during the initial episode and any subsequent recurrences of the disease.

Let me amplify this, because it is a fundamentally important point. During periods of latency, when the virus is lying dormant in nerve tissue, transmission cannot occur. People can go about their lives and fully engage in affectionate and intimate behavior without having to worry about spreading herpes. It simply can't happen. People with herpes are infectious only during periods of active viral recurrences. The first sign of reactivation, then, is an early-warning signal telling you to employ caution and modify your behavior in order not to expose anyone else. Let's look at this more closely, because there may be some confusion about *when* a recurrence is actually in progress.

From the point of view of prevention, reactivation begins with the prodrome. This term describes the sensation that many people experience for several hours or, in some cases, two or more days before the first visible sore reemerges. Why should we care about the prodrome? Simply because that early tingling, itching feeling is not only the first warning sign of an impending recurrence of the virus but may also be an infectious state itself.

During the prodrome the virus is active within the body —cells are being attacked and taken over by the virus. As more cells are invaded and more viruses produced, the tissue destruction increases until the characteristic ulcers appear. But in those first few hours before the development of sores, plenty of active viruses are present just beneath the surface of the skin, enough to constitute an infectious condition. The prodrome, therefore, should be regarded as the beginning of the contagious period.

Learning to recognize the prodrome at the earliest possible moment is a great aid in preventing the spread of herpes. For many, the sensation is obvious and easily identified. For others, the feeling is so subtle that it may be overlooked. Sharpening your sensitivity to what is taking place in your body can enable you to recognize even the faintest indication of a prodrome. For those who have yet to acquire the skill, here is a list of the words and phrases used by many of my patients to describe it. See if one or more of them don't stir up some sense of recognition:

A tingling sensation
An itch

An intermittent prickly pain

A creeping, crawling feeling

The very end of the pins-and-needles feeling

A dull, pulselike throb

A droning ache

A feeling of pressure

A feeling of movement beneath the surface

A ticlike, "spasmatic" feeling

The touch-sensitive feeling you get before a pimple develops

In some cases, the prodrome is accompanied by mild tenderness and slight swelling in nearby lymph glands. In conjunction with labial herpes, the glands beneath the jaw are affected; in cases of genital herpes, it's usually the glands in the lower abdomen. These symptoms, however, are rare during recurrences. Perceptible lymph-gland activity is generally limited to the first episode of herpes, but if you continue to get such signs before and during recurrences, make use of the information.

Right after the prodrome, the typical lesions of herpes begin to form. They start out as a concentrated, reddish-appearing sore or cluster of sores at the affected site and gradually take on a grayish, moist, blisterlike appearance. They are mildly painful when left alone and may be sharply painful if inadvertently rubbed or touched. These sores are loaded with viruses and are, therefore, highly infectious.

Fortunately, these sores are very difficult to miss, even among women with vaginal herpes. This point is terribly important. There is a myth that women with vaginal herpes find it difficult to practice prevention because, unlike penile and labial sores, vaginal sores can't be seen or felt. Once again, a myth can be proven false. Most women with recurrent genital herpes get vulvar lesions that can be easily seen and readily felt. Dr. Lawrence Corey, the prominent herpes virologist and clinician at the University of Washington

School of Medicine in Seattle, has demonstrated that women with genital herpes rarely have cervical sores (which would be difficult to notice) *without* involvement of vulvar tissue near the exterior of the vagina. To focus attention on the rare case of undetectable cervical infection is to ignore the overwhelming majority of cases in which women can easily recognize their recurrences. Let's bury this myth once and for all.

Obviously, during the period when the sores are in their blisterlike or ulcerative form, viruses are present in abundance and the disease is highly contagious, but this is also true even when scabs develop and healing begins. In his classic study, "The Natural History of Recurrent Herpes Simplex Labialis," Dr. Spotswood L. Spruance and his associates at the University of Utah College of Medicine reported the results of studies proving that it was possible to grow the virus from patients sores at every stage of development, including the crusted-over stage. The only stage during which samples from all patients in the study were uniformly negative (no longer infectious) was after the lesions had healed.

The implication for prevention is clear. Since infectiousness correlates with the presence of active viruses at the surface of skin and mucosal tissue, we must regard the entire recurrent episode, from the first recognition of the prodrome to the point at which the sores are completely healed, as the period of contagiousness and the time to practice prevention.

Preventive Behavior

There's no magic to preventing the spread of herpes. In fact, prevention is simple and direct—so direct that I'm going to tell you all you will probably ever need to know about it by selecting the questions my patients invariably ask and answering them briefly.

Q. If I feel the sensations of a recurrence coming up on my lip, what should I do?

A. Don't kiss *anyone*—not your husband or wife, not your boyfriend or girlfriend, not your kids, your friends, your boss, anyone.

Q. By kiss, you mean a deep kiss, right?

A. Wrong—any kind of kiss, big, little, passionate, casual, deep, shallow, or otherwise. Any time your lips touch someone else's mouth, cheek, neck, hands, or any other body part, that's a kiss, and that's what you should not do.

Q. What about when my spouse and I kiss unconsciously in our sleep?

A. If you're serious about prevention and you know that you snuggle up and kiss in your sleep, one option is to sleep separately until the sores are fully healed. If you can't do that, try putting a pillow between your heads, as sort of a kissing barrier. Or try switching sides of the bed for the duration of the episode so that you tend to turn away from your mate. It will take a while before you get comfortable turning the other way, and by then the sores should be gone.

Q. What about my baby, who sometimes touches my face and lips?

A. If your child's movements are too erratic or quick to predict and control, don't chance it. Enjoy him or her at arm's-length until your sores have healed.

Q. What if, despite my best efforts, I accidentally kiss someone?

A. Have that person wash the part that's been kissed with soap and water as soon as possible. The virus doesn't like soap. This may help if the virus hasn't already invaded cells.

Q. What about inanimate objects such as toothbrushes, drinking glasses, eating utensils, plates, pens, doorknobs, and the like?

A. As mentioned several times, the virus can't

survive outside the body; therefore, in general,
don't worry about inanimate objects, especially
objects you normally don't place in your
mouth. Normal washing of glasses, forks, knives,
spoons, and plates after use is sufficient. The
only caution I would give is to avoid sharing
them and toothbrushes while you have the
sores.

Q. Is it possible to contract herpes from a toilet
seat?

A. In general, toilet seats represent no more of a
threat than other inanimate objects, with one
exception: if genital sores are at the "weeping"
stage and some of the exudate gets on the toilet
seat, it's best to wash it off to protect the next
person. Keep in mind, though, that after a short
time any viruses that may have been deposited
will decompose anyway.

Q. Is there any similar rule like "don't kiss" for
people with genital herpes?

A. Yes, the obvious one: don't have sex until the
sores are all gone.

Q. By sex, you mean sexual intercourse, right?

A. Right, more or less. I mean no sexual
intercourse, but also no sex play, not even
romantic embraces that are likely to place the
other person in contact with the sores.

Q. What about using condoms? Aren't they
protective?

A. Their protective efficacy has not been proven.
The virus is smaller than the pores of a condom,
so it could conceivably pass through. The basic
commonsense rule still stands: no sex.

Q. Does the recommendation of not sleeping with
my spouse apply if I have genital herpes?

A. No, that's not necessary. In a sense, genital
herpes is easier than lip herpes to deal with in
bed. There is no practical way to cover your

lips, but you can wear pajamas. That's what I
would recommend.

Q. Is there anything else I should know about
prevention behavior?

A. You already know it all. You know when herpes
is contagious, what behavior leads to spreading
it, and how to act on this information. That's all
you need. As I have said, preventing herpes is
simple and direct.

Q. One last thing, and this is more of a statement
than a question. All this talk about periods of
contagiousness, infectious agents, and how
conscious I have to be not to give herpes to
someone else makes me feel like I'm
permanently quarantined. I know I shouldn't,
but that's exactly how I feel.

A. You are feeling nothing that many other people
haven't felt before. It's perfectly natural at first
to feel a little uncomfortable about having a
disease that is infectious from time to time and
having to modify your behavior to avoid
spreading it. The whole idea is new and takes a
little getting used to, that's all. But remember,
prevention is no big deal. It's easy to do, and
you'll feel good protecting the people you care
about.

WELLNESS AND OTHERS:
THE PREVENTION IMPERATIVE

At the beginning of this chapter, I said that we have been
unwitting conspirators with nature in perpetuating herpes as
an ongoing human illness. Ignorance about the cause of this
infectious disease and the manner in which it is spread have
understandably led to the problem we face today—not just
an epidemic but, by all measures, a superepidemic of herpes.
Fortunately, this is about to change as ignorance gives way
to awareness.

Take what you have learned in this chapter and use it—now. Start right away. Become the vehicle for change by practicing herpes prevention to the best of your ability. As you are a force in your own wellness, so you are also a principal force in the wellness of others. It's the prevention imperative.

CHAPTER 7

WELLNESS AND BABIES: PREGNANCY, BIRTH, AND INFANCY

In keeping with our orientation toward wellness, this chapter is a simple and direct approach to coping with herpes during and immediately following pregnancy. We will explore the facts surrounding the possible prenatal and postnatal complications of herpes and, more important, we will learn how to minimize the risks of this disease to newborn babies.

Just as we can influence our own health, we can take conscious action to preserve the health of our infants.

THE VULNERABLE INFANT

Few aspects of herpes evoke as much concern as the threat this viral disease poses to the health and welfare of newborns. The herpes simplex virus is so threatening to them because of their underdeveloped natural defense mechanisms, which allow the virus to behave like a virulent pathogen (a dangerous disease-causing germ) instead of the minor annoying parasite it normally is in adults and children past infancy.

By now we are quite familiar with the way our body responds to herpes. Our immune system reacts quickly and with great force to check the advance of the virus in a furious but short-lived battle for control. Thanks to the strength of our natural body defenses, cell and tissue destruction is localized and held to a minimum. The battered virus retreats, our body begins to repair the damage, and in only a week or two all evidence of the battle has been removed.

In the fragile and vulnerable body of an infant, however, the scenario is quite different, for the natural defense mechanisms of a newborn baby are incomplete and immature. To begin with, a child enters the world with only a moderate level of protective circulating antibodies (see Chapter 3 for a full discussion of antibodies), which are transferred from the mother to the child during fetal development. Depending upon their adequacy and quality, the degree of protection these antibodies afford the infant early in life may be marginal. It will take several months, perhaps as long as six months, before the baby will be able to produce his or her own antibodies to augment the maternal supply. In the meantime, the baby's defenses are not up to par.

In addition, other immune factors are lacking in a newborn infant. The defensive actions of macrophages, B-lymphocytes, and T-lymphocytes are generally slower and less ferocious in infants than in older children or adults. (See Chapter 3 for a full discussion of cellular immune factors.) This is because they have yet to be sensitized by encounters with their natural enemies, disease organisms like the virus. (See Chapter 4 for details on sensitization.)

The combined effect of these antibody and cellular deficiencies in the immune system causes the newborn to be a relatively unprotected target for the first several months of life. Fortunately, however, infection with the herpes simplex virus does not happen very often in newborns.

Drs. John W. Larsen, Jr., and John H. Grossman, III, coeditors of the *Perinatal Infection Newsletter,* report that between one and five cases of herpes in newborns are observed per 10,000 live births. This estimated case rate translates to between 300 and 1,500 infant infections each year. The National Institutes of Health, however, suggests the case rate to be lower. In the 1979 Task Force Report on Viral Infections, cases of infant herpes were estimated at between 100 and 1,000 per year.

On the basis on these approximations, herpes in newborn babies ranks somewhere between congenital rubella (less than 100 cases are reported each year) and infant cytomegalovirus infection (CMV causes moderate to severe brain damage in 3,000 babies each year). Considering that there are approximately 3 million live births annually, infant herpes is hardly a major epidemic. Sadly, however, it happens; and, sadder still, Drs. Larsen and Grossman fear that its incidence could increase in the future. They base their sobering concern on the fact that the greater the incidence of herpes among women of childbearing age, the greater will be the possibility of infant herpes. And, according to all reliable indicators, herpes is spreading fastest among men and women between the ages of 15 and 35, which, for women, is the period just before and during the peak childbearing years.

Whether or not the incidence of herpes among newborns increases, decreases, or stabilizes, as far as I am concerned every case is one too many, for few diseases can be as destructive or tragic.

FROM MOTHER TO BABY

Transmission of herpes to newborn babies usually happens in one of two ways. Most commonly, the infant contracts the virus during birth. If the mother has an active outbreak of genital herpes at or near the time of delivery, any viruses present in sores or vaginal secretions may enter the baby as it passes the birth canal. The baby can also contract the virus after birth if kissed by someone who has active lip herpes; this method is less common but still leads to infection. So babies, like adults, contract herpes in the time-honored way —as a result of some form of direct contact with the virus.

Regardless of how the baby becomes infected, chances are that the disease will run a predetermined course. The two possible patterns of development in newborn children are well documented: general infection, which usually proves fatal, and local infection, which, although not usually fatal, can leave the child with permanent brain damage.

General infection occurs in approximately two-thirds of all cases, and it is the most severe form of the disease. Since the virus encounters very little resistance in an infant's body, cell-to-cell spread is rapid and extensive. After a short time, usually within twelve hours to a few days, the unchallenged viruses spill over into the bloodstream and are disseminated to all parts of the child's body, a condition known as *viremia*. Vital organs, including the liver, kidneys, spleen, stomach, adrenal glands, lungs, and brain, come under attack, and before long—usually within a week—over 80 percent of the babies die. The children who survive usually suffer severe brain damage. Only about three children in 100 actually recover from this massive infection without apparent brain or organ damage.

Local infection occurs in approximately one-third of the babies who contract the virus, and although it rarely leads to death, it does result in some degree of permanent brain damage in over 40 percent of cases. This form of the disease is characterized by herpes sores distributed around the child's mouth, skin, or eyes. When the eyes are involved, there is danger of corneal damage and partial or complete loss of sight.

Overall, the prognosis for infants who contract herpes, regardless of how it develops, is not very encouraging. Roughly two-thirds die and more than half of the survivors suffer some form of sensory impairment or brain damage.

Before exploring how to prevent infant herpes, I'd like to deal with an important question that is frequently asked by patients: Can the virus affect the baby while it's still in the womb?

The answer is yes, but let me emphasize that it is an extremely rare occurrence. Transplacental infection of a developing fetus could conceivably take place as a result of viremia in the mother, but herpes in adults is usually local and self-limiting; the virus almost never enters the circulating blood supply. In those rare cases where the developing fetus does become infected, miscarriage is the usual outcome; in a sense, nature takes care of its own and doesn't let the pregnancy continue.

PROTECTING YOUR BABY: PRENATAL AND POSTNATAL PREVENTION

The facts surrounding herpes in newborns are promising in one major regard: since transmission is nearly always by direct exposure at or shortly after birth rather than by intrauterine means, infant herpes, like adult herpes, is nearly 100 percent preventable. When I tell prospective mothers this statistic, they sometimes react with incredulity. Following are the questions they ask; the answers speak for themselves.

Q. If I have genital herpes and become pregnant, what should I do?

A. Tell your obstetrician about your herpes. Even if the subject has been discussed at some time in the past, don't assume your doctor remembers. Bring it up again. It is an important part of your medical history, particularly if you are pregnant.

Q. What will my doctor do with this information?

A. If you've never had your infection confirmed by a special culture test (most patients haven't), one of the first things your doctor will do is tell you to be on the lookout for any signs of a recurrence and to come back the instant you notice one. At that point, a specimen will be taken and tested just to make sure that the symptoms you exhibit are those caused by herpes.

Q. What else will my doctor do?

A. Your doctor will probably seek your help in establishing your due date as accurately as possible and question you in great detail about your pattern of recurrences. The more that is

known about how frequently you get them,
exactly where they recur, whether or not you
can recognize your prodrome, and how long
you generally take to heal, the better able your
doctor will be to make good judgments and
provide help if it is needed.

Q. After all that, what else will happen?

A. For most of the remainder of your pregnancy,
you'll follow the standard prenatal procedures.
You will be counseled about how to take care of
yourself in areas such as rest and diet, and you'll
get your routine prenatal exams. The only
difference might be that your doctor may ask
you to come in every time you have a
recurrence.

Q. What about lovemaking? Will that be
prohibited?

A. Generally not. With only two exceptions, the
same rules that always apply during pregnancy
will apply to you.

Q. What are they?

A. As mentioned in Chapter 5, vigorous
intercourse can sometimes lead to recurrence.
If this is true in your case, you'll be cautioned
to be more moderate and to use extra
lubrication. Your doctor might even suggest
that you not take any chances and practice
abstinence during the last four to six weeks
before your due date. The second exception
relates to your spouse. If he has either an initial
infection or a recurrence during the last four to
six weeks of your pregnancy, intercourse should
be avoided so that he doesn't pass the virus to
you.

Q. What will happen as I near term?

A. Anywhere from two to four weeks prior to your
expected due date, your doctor will probably
want to examine you on a regular basis, possibly
weekly. Cultures may be taken even though

nothing appears to be wrong. And you will be told to be meticulously observant and report any prodrome or recurrence the moment you notice it.

Q. What if my doctor finds nothing wrong?

A. If you haven't noticed anything yourself, and if your exams and cultures confirm that nothing is wrong, it's full speed ahead for a routine vaginal delivery and a healthy baby.

Q. What if my herpes recurs near my due date?

A. It depends on how near your due date it happens and how quickly you can be expected to heal. If, for example, you get a recurrence three weeks before you are due and your recurrences generally heal in ten days, your doctor may decide there is a good chance it will be over by the time you're expected to deliver. Your progress will be monitored closely, and if you heal on schedule and your cultures are negative at term, a normal vaginal delivery would seem in order. If you don't heal on schedule, or if signs of labor come earlier than expected, your doctor probably won't want to risk a vaginal delivery. Obviously, if a recurrence develops so close to your expected due date that there is little if any chance of full recovery at term, a vaginal delivery won't be risked.

Q. Let's say that, for any of the above reasons, I can't deliver vaginally. What then?

A. It is for just this eventuality that you and your doctor have taken all the precautions. If it is found that vaginal delivery might expose the emerging infant to the virus, your doctor will arrange to deliver your child by Caesarean section prior to the rupture of fetal membranes. This will prevent the baby from becoming infected, and that's the goal.

Q. What about afterward?

A. It depends. If you still have sores after the baby comes, just make sure that the child doesn't touch them and that you don't touch your baby if you've touched your sores. It's also a good practice to wash your hands thoroughly with soap and water before handling the infant. Once you are completely healed, there's no longer any threat.

Q. So far you've only mentioned genital herpes. What about labial herpes?

A. The same rules apply. Avoid placing the baby in contact with the sores and wash your hands thoroughly before handling him or her. This also applies to anyone else in your family who may have lip herpes during the first four months or so of the baby's life. Keep a safe distance during a recurrence. Of course, even after the baby is no longer an infant, you should avoid giving him or her the infection. Prevention is for now and forever: you never want to spread herpes if you can help it.

Q. You make it seem as if infant herpes never has to happen.

A. That's right, and that's the real tragedy of infant herpes. Although we still haven't realized our 100 percent prevention goal, we're on our way. As people become more cognizant of their power to prevent infant herpes and more willing to tell their doctors about their condition, more and more infant herpes will be prevented. Eventually, it might not exist at all. How's that for a goal?

CHAPTER 8

HERPES AND CANCER: FACT OR FICTION?

In recent years, no aspect of herpes has stirred up as much controversy, provoked as much public concern, or received as much media exposure as the possible link between genital herpes in women and the development of cervical cancer. How real is the link? How much evidence supports it? How much importance should we place on it? What can a woman do about it?

Finding answers to these and other important questions is the focus of this chapter. In the search for answers, some knowledge of the phenomenon of cancer is necessary. We will take a look at the medical observations and research findings that relate viruses to cancerous changes in cells. We will explore what first brought herpes to the attention of scientists and examine what subsequent studies have revealed. Through our discussion of how herpes and cancer fit together, every woman will be able to learn what she can do to safeguard her health.

THE PHENOMENON OF CANCER

In their book *Getting Well Again,* Dr. O. Carl Simonton, Stephanie Matthews-Simonton, and James Creighton offer a basic explanation of what cancer is:

A cancer begins with a cell that contains incorrect genetic information so that it is unable to perform its intended function. This cell may receive the incorrect information because it has been exposed to harmful substances or chemicals or damaged by other external causes, or simply because in the process of constantly reproducing billions of cells the body will occasionally make an imperfect one. If this cell reproduces other cells with the same incorrect genetic makeup, then a tumor begins to form composed of a mass of these imperfect cells. Normally, the body's defenses, the immune system, would recognize these cells and destroy them. At a minimum, they would be walled off so they could not spread.

In the case of malignant cells, sufficient cellular changes take place so that they reproduce rapidly and begin to intrude on adjoining tissue. Whereas there is a form of "communication" between normal cells that prevents them from overreproducing, the malignant cells are sufficiently disorganized so that they do not respond to the communication of the cells around them and they begin to reproduce recklessly. The body normally destroys them. But if it does not, the mass of faulty cells, the tumor, may begin to block proper functioning of body organs, either by expanding to the point that it puts physical pressure on other organs, or by replacing enough healthy cells in an organ with malignant cells so that the organ is no longer able to function.

Clearly, then, cancer is not some dark, mysterious, one-dimensional force that invades our bodies and takes over. Rather, it is the product of a series of interrelated biologic events. An abnormal cell appears, immune defenses fail to destroy it, the defect is passed on as the cell divides, and— if the factors that control overreproduction no longer govern the defective cell—the resulting mass becomes a cancerous tumor. And, as Dr. Simonton has noted, among the other situations that provoke the appearance of abnormal cells, occasionally a cell is damaged as a consequence of viral invasion.

THE VIRAL ROLE IN CANCER

The concept that viruses may play a role in the development of some forms of cancer is not new. For over seventy years scientists have been studying—both in nature and in the laboratory—the ability of certain viruses to induce tumors in animals.

As far back as 1908, two Danish scientists—V. Ellerman and O. Bang—discovered that avian leukosis (a form of leukemia in fowl) was transmitted by a virus. In 1911, another scientist, Peyton Rous of the Rockefeller Institute for Medical Research, demonstrated that sarcoma (a form of cancer in chickens) was also transmitted by a virus. Since then, many more instances of tumors and cancers in animals have been uncovered in which viruses have been proven to cause the cell abnormalities. Leukemia in cats, for instance, is known to be caused by a virus; so is kidney cancer in frogs, lymphoid cancer in chickens (Marek's disease, resembling Hodgkin's disease in people), and mammary cancer in mice.

As scientists learned more about the link between viruses and some animal cancers, it became increasingly obvious that not all viruses were tumor- or cancer-causing. Two major groups of viruses emerged as the most suspect—the retroviruses (also known as oncoviruses), which are responsible for cat, bird, mouse, and monkey tumors, and the herpesviruses (the animal varieties), which are responsible for kidney cancer in frogs and lymphoid cancer in chickens. When scientists began to search for similar instances of virus-induced cancers in humans, it's no wonder that they focused on retroviruses and herpesviruses.

Of these two families of viruses, the evidence linking some of the herpesviruses with human cancers seems to be far clearer and more compelling than the evidence surrounding retroviruses. In fact, herpesviruses are considered the prime candidates as possible viral causes of human cancers, and, among them, the Epstein-Barr virus is the most eligible.

You may recall our characterization of the Epstein-Barr virus (EBV) as one of the five herpesviruses known to infect humans and to be the causative agent of infectious mononucleosis. It now seems our relationship with EBV may be considerably more important.

In 1958, Dr. Denis P. Burkitt, an English surgeon working at Makerere University in Uganda, described an unusual form of neck cancer among African children. The disease, now called Burkitt's lymphoma, was marked by rapid malignant growth of lymphoid tissues, with tumor size doubling every one to two days. For obvious reasons, the disease proved fatal in a short period of time. Dr. Burkitt's interest in studying this previously undescribed form of cancer took him throughout Africa and brought him into contact with hundreds of patients and their families. On the basis of the data he collected, Burkitt surmised that one or more infectious agents either caused or precipitated this common form of childhood cancer in Africa.

In 1964, medical researchers studying Burkitt's lymphoma at Middlesex Hospital in London made an important discovery. M. A. Epstein, B. G. Achong, and Y. M. Barr were examining biopsy specimens of the neck tumors under an electron microscope when they observed, inside the cells, particles of the herpesvirus that today bears their name.

Over the next eight years, scientists throughout the world cooperated to establish that the Epstein-Barr virus and Burkitt's lymphoma were related, but not always in a direct manner. For while EBV has been demonstrated to cause cancerous cell defects, not everyone who becomes infected with it develops this form of cancer. In fact, in the United States and other countries where the standard of living is high, Burkitt's lymphoma is virtually nonexistent even though the virus is quite widespread. In African children, the appearance of this cancer after viral invasion was caused by the suppression of the natural body defenses as a result of malaria, which is prevalent in the parts of Africa where Burkitt's lymphoma is found. The defective cells survived and grew into tumors.

This link between one herpesvirus—the EBV—and a form of cancer served to fuel a speculative fire that other herpesviruses, including herpes simplex, might be implicated in some human cancers as well—a fire, it turns out, that had been burning for some time.

HERPES SIMPLEX AND CANCER

Around the turn of the century, Dr. H. N. Vineberg, a gynecologist in New York City, diagnosed cervical cancer in one of his patients. This alone was not remarkable, for he had seen this condition dozens of times before. What seemed unusual to him, however, was that this particular woman was Jewish, and Dr. Vineberg had rarely encountered cervical cancer among his Jewish patients.

Intrigued by his diagnosis, Dr. Vineberg was motivated to dig deeper, and began the arduous process of searching through twenty years of medical records to find some clues. At the end of this process, he succeeded in documenting that, in fact, cervical cancer was twenty times less frequent among his Jewish patients than among his non-Jewish patients.

Determining what this finding meant presented a problem for Dr. Vineberg. The factors which, in 1905, were believed by the medical profession to be associated with cervical cancer—impoverished living conditions, early marriage, and many pregnancies—were quite common among his Jewish patients, who then lived primarily in overcrowded slum sections of New York. Why, then, wasn't cervical cancer more common among this group of women than his study indicated? With little more than his own data and his power of deductive reasoning to guide him, Dr. Vineberg finally concluded that three factors unique to the Jewish community must be responsible for the lower incidence of cervical cancer among Jewish women: heredity (intermarriage then was rare), traditional dietary customs, and the ritualized practice among Jewish people of abstaining from sexual relations during a woman's menstrual period.

Over thirty years later, in 1936, another inquisitive physician, Dr. A. S. Handley, observed a similar disparity in cervical cancer rates among his female patients in the Fiji Islands. Dr. Handley found that his Moslem patients developed the condition much less frequently than his Hindu patients and set out to determine why.

Aware of Dr. Vineberg's earlier speculations and findings with regard to cervical cancer among Jewish women, Dr. Handley began searching for some factor common to Jews and Moslems that might serve to explain both disparities. With heredity clearly the wrong avenue of pursuit, and discounting the role of diet in this form of cancer, Dr. Handley turned his attention to ritual practices shared by both peoples and indeed found a link: the traditional rite of male circumcision, practiced universally by Moslems and Jews but only rarely by Hindus and people of other religious backgrounds. This difference, Dr. Handley suggested, served to validate both his and Vineberg's observations, and he concluded that the risks of cervical cancer were reduced among women whose husbands had been circumcised. But how? Another thirty or so years were to pass before these questions would begin to get answered.

By the 1960s, medical researchers were conducting studies throughout the world to gather as much information as possible about cervical cancer. These studies involved thousands of women with and without cervical cancer from every conceivable social, economic, and cultural stratum.

Between 1963 and 1966, cancer investigators at Emory University in Atlanta and Baylor College of Medicine in Houston, in cooperation with scientists from Great Britain, conducted extensive comparative studies involving thousands of cervical-cancer patients, including nuns and prostitutes. These investigations showed that cervical cancer was most prevalent among prostitutes, almost nonexistent among nuns, and relatively more frequent among women who began sex early in life and had many different sexual partners than among women who began sex later and had only one sexual partner. Since Dr. Handley's hypothesis about sexual exposure to circumcised or uncircumcised males failed to explain these differences, scientists analyzed the data extensively to identify some factor that would.

And they did find a common element—the patterns indicated that sex itself was the prime correlate. Scientists knew something was missing. They didn't believe that sexual intercourse alone was the answer but speculated that some undetermined factor linked sexual activity—particularly multiple-partner sexual activity—with the risk of cervical cancer. As more investigations were completed and more information became available, it became increasingly clear that cervical cancer was related to and possibly even transmitted by sex.

In Puerto Rico, Dr. I. Martinez examined the wives of nearly 900 men with skin cancer of the penis and detected cervical cancer among eight of them. Was cancer being transmitted? Dr. Martinez couldn't be certain about this, because coincidence could easily explain his finding. Interestingly, however, Dr. Martinez examined the wives of the 889 men who did not have penile cancer and found not one case of cervical cancer.

And at the University of Maryland's medical school, Dr. Irving Kessler came up with the most interesting finding of all. After examining a cross-section of several thousand women, he found cervical cancer to be three or four times as prevalent among women married to men whose *former* wives had had cervical cancer as among women married to men who had not been married before or whose former wives had not had cervical cancer. In an article in *New Times* magazine discussing his own findings as well as those of other researchers into cervical cancer, Dr. Kessler wrote: "In every study done, the cancer has followed a venereal pattern. The association between sexual intercourse and cervical cancer is as well documented as that between cholesterol and heart disease, if not better."

Because sexual transmission of cervical cancer was strongly suspected, investigators began speculating that some infectious agent might be the culprit. Attempts were made to link cervical cancer with syphilis and gonorrhea, the two most prominent sexually transmitted diseases of the time, but no connection could be established with either one. And then, aware of the newly discovered association between the Epstein-Barr virus—a herpesvirus—and Burkitt's lymphoma, the researchers turned to another herpesvirus

that was becoming increasingly prevalent as a sexually transmitted agent: the herpes simplex virus.

When medical researchers attempted to relate the incidence and patterns of herpes to those of cervical cancer they
finally struck pay dirt. In study after study conducted by the
most prominent investigators, strong correlations were cited
between cervical cancer and prior infection with genital
herpes. Dr. W. E. Rawls, at the Baylor College of Medicine,
found evidence that genital herpes was twice as frequent
among cervical-cancer patients as among matched controls
without cervical cancer. Dr. Andre J. Nahmias of the Emory
University School of Medicine found genital herpes to be
three times as common among women with cervical cancer
as in matched controls. Tests conducted in West Virginia,
Chicago, Baltimore, and Boston all yielded the same results:
evidence of genital herpes was found two to three times
more often among cervical-cancer patients than among
women without the condition.

With all indications pointing to the herpes simplex virus as
the elusive, long-sought factor in cervical cancer, Dr.
Nahmias wrote in *Today's Health* magazine that women
who suffer genital herpes infections are eight times more
likely to develop cervical cancer than those without herpes.
Commenting on the preliminary results of a study involving
1,500 women—900 with herpes and 600 without—Dr.
Nahmias predicted that 6 percent of the women with genital
herpes would develop cervical cancer within five years.

Despite the accretion of evidence clearly relating genital
herpes and cancer of the cervix, two questions had to be
answered before the nature of the relationship could be understood. First, does infection with the virus precede or follow the development of cervical cancer? Second, is the virus
capable of transforming a normal cell into the defective,
cancerous cell?

The chicken-or-the-egg question—which happens first,
contracting herpes or developing cervical cancer—is fundamental to any attempt to define the relationship. Obviously,
if the development of cervical cancer precedes infection
with the herpesvirus, the possibility that herpes causes or

even induces cancerous cell changes is not viable. The answer came in 1970 when Dr. Laure Aurelian of the Johns Hopkins School of Medicine demonstrated that infection with herpes preceded the earliest identifiable states of cervical cancer. While this finding didn't establish a definitive cause-and-effect relationship, it didn't preclude one, either.

The question of whether herpes simplex viruses can convert normal cells into cells with malignant properties was answered in 1971 by Dr. Fred Rapp and his associates at the Hershey Medical Center of the Pennsylvania State University, who demonstrated that the virus could transform normal hamster cells into cancer cells. Since then, the virus has been shown to cause cancerous defects in the cells of chickens and mice, and even in human cells in tissue culture.

The answers to these questions, together with the statistical finding that cervical cancer is many times more common among women with genital herpes than among women with no history of the disease, led to the all-important question: Does genital herpes cause cervical cancer?

The current view is that, in spite of all the evidence brought to light by medical researchers, there is still no proven cause-and-effect relationship between genital herpes and cervical cancer. What *has* been proven beyond any doubt is that the virus is a significant risk factor in the transformation of normal cells into defective ones. This does not mean that women with genital herpes should expect to develop cervical cancer later in life but that their risk of developing the condition appears to be six or more times greater than if they weren't infected with the virus.

From a practical point of view, the knowledge that genital herpes is a risk factor can be put to good use. Since a routine PAP test once a year can minimize the possibilities of cervical cancer in any woman, women who have a history of genital herpes are advised to receive PAP tests every six months. This is only twice as often as normal, and the benefits far outweigh any minor inconveniences. The test, which involves taking a painless scraping from the cervix and examining it under a microscope, will reveal cervical-tissue abnormalities and cell changes at the earliest possible moment.

When such changes are detected early, the treatment is simple (it's done in the doctor's office), painless, inexpensive, and effective in preventing the abnormal cells from developing into a true cancer.

CHAPTER 9

———

SOME ADDITIONAL CONCERNS: KERATITIS, ENCEPHALITIS, AND IMMUNOSUPPRESSION

———

We've come a long way in our exploration of herpes and the development of a wellness approach to coping with it. We've seen how a positive attitude, healthful behavior, and conscious attempts to reduce stress and practice good hygiene may minimize the problems of recurrent disease. We've learned how important prevention is and how to avoid spreading the disease to others. We've come to realize that pregnancy and childbirth need not be complicated by herpes so long as we are aware of the possible risks and take steps to avoid them. And we've concluded that even the risk of cervical cancer can be lessened by the precaution of getting a PAP test every six months.

In all these discussions, we have been able to analyze complicated and sometimes disturbing aspects of the disease and yet come away feeling hopeful and optimistic because in each area there are opportunities for self-help and the achievement of wellness. Replacing incorrect mythical beliefs with objective realities, we have probed and evaluated our belief systems and our attitudes, and where necessary we have altered them to better accommodate new information, greater insights, and a growing commitment to improving ourselves. In so doing we have identified pathways that will lead us to health, wellness, and a life as free as possible from the burden of herpes.

In this chapter, we are going to follow a somewhat different model. There are three dimensions of herpes that don't quite fit into a self-help approach because there are so few opportunities to alter them, so instead of educating, I will be informing. The subject matter of this chapter, although potentially threatening, has not been germane to the development of a wellness approach, and in order to gain a proper perspective on this information it was first necessary to obtain more knowledge about herpes, which the preceding chapters have provided. I have chosen to include this material because I believe you have the right to be aware of everything that is known to date about herpes.

GAINING THE PROPER PERSPECTIVE

Mumps, measles, chicken pox, and influenza—do we consider them dangerous, debilitating or life-threatening? Hardly. But did you know that each of these very common diseases can be life-threatening?

This is true. In 1974, there were reports of six deaths from mumps, twenty from measles, 106 from chicken pox, and over 2,000 from influenza. In comparison to the tens of millions of cases that occur each year (and during a year in which there is a flu epidemic, the number could easily exceed 100 million), slightly more than 2,000 deaths doesn't evoke a sense of terror.

Our attitude toward these diseases is approximately the same with respect to complications and possible lifelong disabilities. Even though they occur, they are so infrequent that worrying about them would be inappropriate and serve no purpose.

What does all this have to do with herpes? It's a gentle reminder to keep your sense of proportion with respect to what's worth worrying about and what isn't as we look at three special problems associated with herpes: herpes keratitis (eye herpes), herpes encephalitis (brain infection), and complications that could result among immunosuppressed persons. As we will see, even though these problems occur, and even though they are quite dangerous when they do, they are so rare that worrying about them is not only unwarranted but detrimental to a wellness orientation.

HERPES KERATITIS

Herpes keratitis, also called ocular herpes, is a herpes simplex virus infection in the eye. The parts of the eye usually involved are the conjunctival membranes, which line the inner surface of the eyelids and extend over the surface of the eye, and the cornea, the transparent external part of the eyeball behind which are the iris (which opens and closes in response to changes in light) and the pupil (the aperture in the center of the iris).

Since doctors aren't required by law to report cases of herpes keratitis, the only data available are estimates made by government agencies and researchers in the field; unfortunately, however, the disparity is great. In its 1979 Task Force Report on Viral Infections, the National Institute of Allergy and Infectious Diseases of the National Institutes of Health estimated 500,000 cases of herpes keratitis each year. Dr. Herbert Blough, a prominent herpes researcher at the Scheie Eye Institute in Philadelphia, estimates 50,000 to 100,000 cases a year. Most other researchers and at least one pharmaceutical firm engaged in herpes research offer a variety of estimates scattered between these two extremes (50,000 to 500,000). The average is around 300,000, but no one can pinpoint the figure with any certainty. I am more inclined to accept the lower estimates; ocular herpes is less common than the larger numbers would indicate. The infection may be caused in one of two ways: by autoinoculation or by neurogenic spread. There is no way to gauge which method is most common, because the statistics do not distinguish between the two types.

Autoinoculation—self-transfer of the virus into the eye—is the direct result of touching an active sore and then inadvertently rubbing or touching one or both eyes. It can also result from the use of saliva as wetting agent for moistening contact lenses during an outbreak of lip herpes. Fortunately, we've seen that by consciously trying not to touch your sores, washing your hands after each accidental contact with a lesion and before touching your eyes, and not using saliva as a wetting agent for contact lenses, you can prevent an outbreak of herpes keratitis.

In addition to self-transfer, the virus may gain entry into the eye neurogenically. As noted in our discussion of recurrences, during the latent phase of lip herpes the virus lies dormant in a nerve cluster called the trigeminal ganglia. Reactivation results when viruses track from this cluster along nerve pathways back to the lips, its customary course. Infrequently, however, instead of following its usual path along nerves leading to the lips, the virus migrates along nerve fibers that lead into the eye and its surrounding tissue. Neurogenic spread is accidental and there is no way to prevent it from happening.

However the virus gains entry into the eye, once it is there the infection progresses in the same way for both types. The first symptom a person with ocular herpes is likely to notice is that irritating feeling of having something in the eye. This early sensation may not be accompanied by any visible signs, particularly if the affected part of the eye is the conjunctival lining under the eyelid. Photophobia (sensitivity to light) and pain may be present, but often these symptoms don't develop until later.

As the infection continues to develop, the conjunctival tissue lining the eyeball, and the cornea directly behind it, may come under attack once the outer surface has been breached. Marked irritation, photophobia, and pain become evident, and an inflammation reminiscent of pink-eye may be noticed. In addition, visible herpes lesions may appear on the surface of the eyeball. The onslaught of the virus may be confined to these outermost parts of the eye, or it may run deeper.

By this time the body has begun to fight back against the virus. Inflammation, irritation, lesions, and sloughing off of fluids are pronounced. Immune defenses eventually gain the upper hand and the eye starts to heal, but the damage to the cornea or deeper tissue may be so extensive that vision may be partially or fully impaired. This may be compounded by scar tissue that replaces the normally transparent cornea.

The statistics associated with the clinical course of ocular herpes are as ill-defined as the incidence estimates. For instance, the duration of infection is highly variable. The frequency of mild eye infections (those limited to the conjunctival tissues) as compared to more extensive involvement of the cornea and deeper tissue is unknown, and there are only crude estimates as to how often the problem resolves itself spontaneously without any damage (this does happen in some cases). The only statistic that is relatively well defined is the result of the infections; according to Dr. Blough, ocular herpes is the most frequent cause of infectious blindness in the United States today. (Glaucoma is the most frequent cause of blindness overall, but it doesn't involve an infectious agent.) He estimates that between 15,000 and 20,000 persons lose their sight because of herpes each year.

Ocular herpes is further complicated by an additional problem: recurrences. According to Dr. Deborah Pavan-Langston, a professor of ophthalmology at Harvard Medical School and a clinician at the Massachusetts Eye and Ear Infirmary, once the virus attacks the eye it can recur there repeatedly, just as in other parts of the body. She estimates that 50 percent of the cases recur, which parallels Dr. Blough's estimate of 50 to 75 percent, and both agree that if it weren't for recurrences, eye specialists would have an easier time dealing with ocular herpes.

This brings us to the one bit of good news about herpes infections of the eye—they can be treated. At present two antiviral agents to treat ocular herpes are licensed for widespread use in the United States: Stoxil and Vira-A. Both are used topically in the eye, and both interfere with the progress of the virus. When a case of ocular herpes is caught before there is major damage to the eye, these products have been shown to halt the infection and totally protect vision. Unfortunately, however, they aren't cures, and each time there is a recurrence the treatment has to be repeated.

All of this is to say that ocular herpes will probably not be a problem for you. Your insurance policy is to avoid transferring the virus into your eyes by meticulously following the rules of prevention summarized in this chapter and presented in detail in Chapter 5. And should you develop one of the early symptoms of eye infection, go to an ophthalmologist at once. The condition is easy to diagnose and treat, but treatment must be started at the earliest possible moment.

HERPES ENCEPHALITIS

A second possible complication is herpes encephalitis—infection of the brain—the most serious of the three but, fortunately, relatively uncommon. As is true of herpes keratitis, doctors aren't required by law to report herpes encephalitis and therefore the exact incidence is unknown. Estimates made by the National Institute of Allergy and Infectious Diseases, Dr. Andre J. Nahmias of the Emory University School of Medicine, and Dr. Bernard Roizman of the University of Chicago Pritzker School of Medicine range from a low of 100 cases to a high of 4,000 cases annually. Despite the large variance, both estimates indicate that the problem is slight in comparison to the tens of millions of people who harbor the herpesvirus.

Herpes encephalitis is unknown among people with genital herpes, as it is associated exclusively with cases of oral, labial, and facial herpes. The only way herpes encephalitis can occur is neurogenically, when the virus moves from the trigeminal ganglia along nerve pathways leading into the brain. (This can't happen in genital herpes because the trigeminal ganglia isn't involved.) And just as ocular herpes resulting from neurogenic spread is a biologic accident, so is herpes encephalitis. No one really understands why the virus occasionally migrates to the brain instead of following its usual path back to the lips, mouth, or face.

The symptoms and consequences of herpes encephalitis reflect the activity of the virus in the brain. Its earliest symptoms are diffuse, including fever, headaches, changes in personality, speech problems, perceptual difficulties, muscle aches, and general weakness. As the infection progresses and the condition of the patient deteriorates, the symptoms worsen, leading to seizures and, eventually, coma. Spontaneous recovery is rare; infection proves fatal in over 70 percent of the cases, and most of those who do survive are left with permanent brain damage, sometimes so severe as to require institutionalization.

Like herpes active elsewhere in the body, herpes encephalitis follows the now-familiar pattern of cellular invasion and takeover, forced production of new viruses, cell destruction, and cell-to-cell spread. And an immune defense is mounted against the virus in the brain, transforming it into a cellular battlefield. Infected cells are ingested by macrophages, blown apart by antibodies and the complement system, and poisoned by lymphocytes. The crucial difference between herpes in the brain and herpes elsewhere is that the victims of this heated exchange between virus and immune defenders are brain cells, which, unlike skin or mucosal cells, can't be replaced once they are damaged or destroyed.

Depending on the severity of the infection, the amount of brain tissue involved, the part of the brain affected, and the speed and forcefulness of the immune response, brain damage may range from slight to moderate, although in most cases it is profound and, as we have just noted, fatal. To repeat my earlier caution, however, as frightening as herpes encephalitis is, it is quite rare.

What can be done about herpes encephalitis? Until recently, nothing. Then, in August 1977, after five years and $1.2 million worth of development and testing, a breakthrough was reported by a National Institute of Allergy and Infectious Diseases study group headed by Drs. Charles A. Alford and Richard J. Whitely of the University of Alabama.

A new drug, adenine arabinoside (ara-A), had been proven to be highly useful in treating people with herpes encephalitis. Although there was one noteworthy problem, the clinical trials demonstrated that very early administration of ara-A could reduce fatality from 70 percent to zero; furthermore, over 75 percent of the survivors suffered only moderate or, in many cases, no brain damage.

The noteworthy problem was that of time: how *soon* the condition came to the attention of a doctor, how *long* it took to establish a diagnosis, and how *quickly* thereafter treatment was administered. Time is the crucial factor, because once it is ensconced in the brain the virus works rapidly. Partial or complete loss of consciousness occurs about six days after the first appearance of symptoms, an indication of such extensive brain damage that treatment may be futile. The following data reported by Alford and Whitely illustrate the critical impact of time on the outcome of treatment:

Among those patients whose treatment was begun prior to loss of consciousness, all survived; of these, over 40 percent were free of brain damage; 40 percent suffered moderate brain damage; and only 20 percent sustained severe brain damage.

Among those patients whose treatment was not started until after they had reached a semicomatose state, 25 percent died; 50 percent of the survivors sustained severe brain damage, and only the remaining 25 percent recovered fully.

Among those patients whose treatment was not started until after coma had developed, 57 percent died and all the survivors sustained severe brain damage.

You may be wondering why time should be a problem at all with a condition this serious. Wouldn't patients go to their doctors at once? Wouldn't doctors make a diagnosis immediately? Wouldn't treatment be instituted at the earliest possible moment? Ideally, yes—but there are roadblocks to discovery, diagnosis, and treatment at each junction.

The first roadblock is the diffuse and nonspecific nature of the early symptoms of herpes encephalitis. How concerned would you be if you started to run a fever, felt weak, and developed head and muscle aches? How many times have you experienced this exact constellation of symptoms and, without calling a doctor, gone to bed on the assumption you were coming down with a cold or the flu? These are not what you would expect as the obvious and threatening signs of a beginning brain infection. Even some of the more pronounced early symptoms such as personality changes, disorientation, and lethargy might fail to generate enough alarm to cause you to see a doctor at once. Meanwhile, the infection gets worse as each day passes.

The second roadblock is the difficulty a doctor faces in trying to establish a diagnosis. Even if the early signs alarm you sufficiently to see your doctor, a quick diagnosis of herpes encephalitis is not easy to make. Look at the symptoms that must be sifted through: fever, headache, muscle aches, weakness, lethargy—all symptoms of the flu, and 99.9 percent of the time that's exactly what it is. If, in addition to these general symptoms, your personality is sufficiently altered and your disorientation is pronounced enough, your doctor may think about some sort of brain problem. The question is, what kind?

A quick examination, a few questions, and a head injury is ruled out. That leaves a probable brain infection—but, again, what kind? Your doctor hospitalizes you and orders the usual workup, serologic tests, various blood counts, analyses of cerebrospinal fluid, and a variety of brain scans, all necessary but time-consuming procedures. Within a day or two, the results of the tests clearly indicate a brain infection, but there is still no confirmation of what kind. Unfortunately, none of these standard tests is definitive for herpes encephalitis.

Your doctor knows that dealing with a brain infection is a race against time, and although it would be tempting to make an educated guess and institute treatment accordingly, chances are your doctor won't. The wrong treatment wouldn't help, and—worse—it could do some harm.

Your doctor may be forced to employ a test that most physicians hesitate to use, a brain biopsy. This procedure consists of drilling into the skull, inserting a needle, and withdrawing a small portion of brain tissue for laboratory analysis. Brain biopsy is by its very nature an invasive procedure attended by all the usual risks that accompany surgery: infection, reaction to anesthesia, and complications. In addition, doctors don't like to remove even a small amount of brain tissue, because there's no way for the body to replace it.

Ironically, this last-resort test is the only definitive way to confirm a diagnosis of herpes encephalitis, but the reluctance to use it causes a delay in ara-A therapy, which, as we have seen, diminishes in effectiveness with each passing day.

The preceding scenario is not meant to frighten you, but it is a real dilemma faced by even the most skilled and competent physicians. It is summed up very clearly in the following statement from a study on herpes encephalitis conducted at Baylor College of Medicine in Houston by a research team headed by Dr. Larry H. Taber and consisting of several prominent immunologists, neurologists, and microbiologists: "Significant reduction in post-treatment neurological and psychological sequellae will almost certainly require earlier diagnosis. At the present time, the only definitive method for diagnosing HSE [herpes simplex encephalitis] is by brain biopsy demonstration of the virus."

Today many doctors who are reasonably sure they are dealing with herpes encephalitis use ara-A because of its life-saving potential and the time-consuming difficulties in establishing a definitive diagnosis. Their earlier reluctance to use this drug in the absence of a firm diagnosis was based on its newness and on an uncertainty as to its harmful side effects. It is now known to be sufficiently, if not entirely, nontoxic to warrant its use in life-and-death situations; many doctors feel the benefits outweigh the risks and prescribe it as early as possible, even on the basis of clinical diagnosis. The basic feeling is that ara-A is too potent a weapon to ignore.

IMMUNOSUPPRESSION

Immunosuppression is not a complication of herpes in the same sense as keratitis or encephalitis, which are natural and accidental. The complications associated with herpes in an immunosuppressed person are rather the unfortunate results of a new medical therapy: transplant antirejection chemotherapy.

Over a span of just twenty years the technology of organ transplants has been developed and refined to the point where transplants are practical and not unduly difficult. So far, more than 3,000 have been performed; diseased kidneys are the most frequently replaced, but hearts, lungs, livers, and bone marrow are also transplanted.

Transplant technology is truly a modern wonder, and yet problems still exist—not surgical but immunologic problems, specifically those of rejection and the sometimes-tragic results of antirejection therapy. And it turns out that one of the most common problems complicating kidney transplants is reactivation of herpes simplex viruses during antirejection treatment. Let's see what this means.

The immune defense system that so capably protects us from countless infections does so at the molecular level. The attraction of macrophages to germs, the coating action of antibodies, the initiation of the complement reaction, and the deadly pursuit of T-lymphocytes, the so-called killer cells, are all physical and chemical reactions that are mechanistic and automatic. These specialized cells and chemicals are activated only by the antigens on the surface of microbes and other foreign objects that identify them as not belonging in the body. Once provoked by antigens, the immune system behaves like a mindless warrior engaged in a primal battle that ends either in victory over the invader or defeat and death of the host.

To the immune system, anything that doesn't belong in the body is considered to be an invader and is fought—and this includes transplanted organs. This is the rejection phenomenon, which remains the biggest hurdle to overcome in transplants, for the immune defense against a new organ is just as violent and massive as it is against bacterium or virus, and just as lethal. Within twenty-four hours of a transplant, the new organ can be so damaged that it must be removed.

Until medical research devises a way of tricking the immune system into thinking the new organ belongs there, or a means of selectively depressing immune defenses so that they will leave the new organ alone and yet still protect us against microbes, doctors are forced to rely upon a variety of immunosuppressive drugs to prevent rejection. Antilymphocyte globulin and steroids can halt B- and T-lymphocyte function, interrupt antibody production, and curb the development of macrophages. This antirejection therapy can in fact bring about a total cessation in immune response so that the transplanted organ is not attacked—but at what price?

The suppression of natural body defense mechanisms is total. Not only won't the new organ be attacked, *nothing* will be—including any bacteria and viruses to which the patient might be exposed. Immunosuppressed patients are so vulnerable to infection that isolation procedures and sterile techniques are rigidly enforced. At this point even a cold could prove devastating to the patient, who has no defenses to fight it.

But disease organisms may already be present in the patient's body—for example, a herpes simplex virus that is normally held in check by natural defenses. Unopposed by immune factors, the virus is able to reactivate, and—with nothing standing in its way—what would otherwise be a limited foray becomes a rapidly escalating general infection. Sores may develop over a larger surface than usual. Deeper tissues may be involved or, worse, the increasing number of viruses may spill over into the circulating blood supply and be deposited in tissues and organs throughout the body.

Faced with a mounting herpes infection in an immunosuppressed organ-transplant patient, a doctor may have to decide between two equally disturbing choices. If the infection gets bad enough, discontinuing immunosuppressive therapy will give the patient a fighting chance against the virus. The recovery of immune function, however, will greatly increase the likelihood of organ rejection. Continuing antirejection therapy will spare the organ, but the damage caused by the virus may create grave complications and possibly even prove fatal.

These problems are being encountered with increasing frequency because of the epidemic nature of herpes and the proliferation of both transplant technology and antirejection therapy. As of now there are no answers, but research is being carried out to find effective antiviral compounds and to devise ways to selectively alter immune response. If successful, these efforts may provide the solution.

CHAPTER 10

WOULD-BE "CURES": PAST AND PRESENT

Like other chronic diseases that don't respond reliably or predictably to treatment, herpes has inspired us to dream. Patients dream of a cure that will quickly relieve or prevent sores. Doctors dream of a shot, pill, or ointment that will enable them to fulfill their responsibility to herpes patients.

Until very recently, the history of research to find a cure or even an effective treatment for herpes has been littered with dreams. For this chapter I have chosen, from an extensive list of dreams, some that are representative of the approaches that have been tried and a few that you may have heard of and are wondering about. In the next chapter we will look at those dreams that have become reality and those that show even greater promise for the future.

TESTING, TESTING: THE TERMINOLOGY OF EVALUATION

Before we examine any of the treatments, we need to define several scientific terms and concepts related to medical experimentation that provide the evaluative context for new antiviral developments.

The *placebo effect,* a term already encountered in our

brief discussion of the ether experiment in Chapter 4, is a factor that affects all drug testing. You may recall that a placebo is a substance or preparation that simulates the real drug tested but is made from ingredients with no therapeutic value. The word derives from the Latin for "I shall be pleasing," which accurately describes how placebos are used—simply to please patients—and hints at their psychological power: pleased patients recover from illness better than patients who aren't pleased. This is the placebo effect, which may occur as an adjunct to any treatment.

The known power of the placebo effect complicates drug testing. Unless appropriate controls are built into the design of an experiment, it can be exceedingly difficult to measure the true effectiveness of a test drug, since the power of the placebo effect enters into every shot, pill, or ointment given to a patient as an "active ingredient."

A good *study design* weeds out the placebo effect and other complicating variables. The term refers to how an experiment is conducted, how subjects are selected, and to what extent controls are used. Open trials, double-blind placebo-controlled trials, and random double-blind placebo-controlled trials are the study designs most often used.

Open trials are the least definitive design for testing the effect of a possible treatment because no attempt is made to eliminate sample distortion, the placebo effect, investigator bias, or any other undesirable variable. Subjects are selected and enrolled in the study on a first-come, first-serve basis and, therefore, may not be representative of all patients with the illness the drug is designed to cure. Every subject receives not only the test drug but, unavoidably, a liberal dosage of the placebo effect, since the subjects taking the drug hope that it will cure them. The problem here is that we have no way of measuring the placebo effect against the effect of the drug itself. The evaluating investigator, usually someone who is hoping for a successful outcome, may be somewhat less than objective in interpreting the results. The results of open trials are almost always meaningless in definitive scientific terms. Unfortunately, open trials are quite common because they are inexpensive and easy to conduct.

In double-blind placebo-controlled trials, subjects are divided into two groups that are usually matched for age, sex, and medical history; one group is tested with the drug and the other—the control group—is "tested" with a placebo. Neither the investigator nor the subjects know which group has received which drug until the end of the study. This elaborate design effectively controls for the placebo effect and investigator bias, but it nevertheless has one shortcoming: patients are still enrolled as subjects on a first-come, first-serve basis and thus may not be representative of all those who need the drug.

A random double-blind placebo-controlled trial is the most elaborate and definitive design of all. In addition to controls against the placebo effect and investigator bias, the design imposes one other condition: random sampling. The subjects are chosen at random to ensure that the study sample will be highly representative of all people with a similar problem. As you might expect, trials using this design are the most expensive and time-consuming to complete.

If a test drug has been demonstrated to be effective on the basis of a good study design, other researchers must then conduct similar experiments with it. The *reproducibility of results* is a basic requirement in the process of validating a new drug or treatment procedure because the drug will be accepted only if additional trials bear out the original results. This rules out the possibility that the first result was a freak occurrence.

Study designs are worked up for use with both humans and animals. There is a further distinction between experimental observations inside and outside the body. *In vivo* experimentation refers to work done in living organisms, either animals or humans. *In vitro* experimentation refers to work done in glass—a test tube, culture plate, or beaker—usually in a laboratory. Many scientific and medical discoveries have stemmed from preliminary experimentation and observations made in vitro, such as the chemical destruction of a particular germ in a test tube or on a culture plate. Most drugs are developed through in vitro testing, of which Alexander Fleming's accidental discovery that penicillin curbed the growth of bacteria on a culture plate is perhaps the best-known example. Unfortunately, not all in vitro discoveries translate into effective drugs for use with humans because the human body, unlike a test tube, is an intricate web of reactions. Such factors as metabolism, tissue penetration, and undesirable side effects may complicate, diminish, confound, or render impractical the action of a new drug that appears promising in vitro. Thus it is clear that in vitro observations must be subjected to stringent in vivo experimentation before a drug's effectiveness and safety can be determined.

With the preceding concepts clearly in mind, we can evaluate the following would-be cures and treatments in terms of proper experimental design. We will also examine the degree to which claims for effectiveness are supported or refuted by the facts.

IMMUNE STIMULATORS

By this time we are thoroughly familiar with the natural protective activity of the immune system in resisting and fighting the herpes infection. We know that the speed and ferocity with which our immune system responds make a big difference in how ill we get and how often the virus is able to reactivate.

Over forty years ago, at a time when virology was in its infancy and immune mechanisms were not completely understood or even identified, scientists began speculating that if some way could be found to rev up the immune system—shorten its reaction time and increase its intensity factor—herpes might be reduced in severity and possibly even cured. Several attempts to do just this have been tried with the substances in two major categories: specific immune stimulators and nonspecific immune stimulators.

Specific Immune Stimulators: Preparations Made from the Virus Itself

The underlying theory that led to the development and testing of herpes simplex virus-specific immune stimulators was the result of scientific observations of the body's immune response to herpes. Immune response—both antibody production specifically targeted against the virus and sensitization of lymphocytes and macrophages to herpes simplex antigens (the surface properties of the virus that mark it for destruction)—is known to be all-important in the body's initial ability to resist the virus. Furthermore, it is known that virus-specific antibodies and sensitizing chemicals are produced and reach high levels in response to active infection. These processes can be measured in blood samples; in previously uninfected persons, scientists observed that chemical concentrations reached very high levels as the active infection proceeded and then receded gradually after the battle was won.

The decreasing concentrations of antibodies and sensitizing chemicals alerted them to the desirability of maintaining the higher levels of these chemicals. Once the active infection had been controlled, the virus had entered a state of latency, and there was no further viral provocation, production of defensive chemicals stopped. Although detectable levels remained for a while, the existing antibodies and sensitizing chemicals eventually decayed.

Scientists then postulated that at some point such a minute concentration of protective chemicals remained that the virus was able to reemerge from latency. If a method could be found to stimulate continued production of virus-specific antibodies and sensitizing chemicals during latency, high concentrations would remain at all times, possibly leading to decreased recurrences or perhaps none.

Various preparations were developed from herpes simplex viruses inactivated either by a chemical called formalin or by heat. Although the inactivated viruses were no longer able to cause disease, they still retained their surface antigens and, therefore, could continue to stimulate the body to produce defensive chemicals.

The earliest testing of this theory was reported in 1938 by Dr. S. F. Frank in the *Journal of Investigative Dermatology.* It was a failure. After multiple injections of a formalin-inactivated herpes simplex virus preparation, Dr. Frank was not able to demonstrate any clear-cut pattern of increased neutralizing chemicals in the blood of test patients. In addition, the majority of patients continued to experience herpes just as they had before receiving the preparation.

The next test came in 1950, when Drs. S. G. Anderson, J. Hamilton, and S. Williams reported on their attempt to prevent primary herpes infection using a formalin-inactivated virus preparation. Their subjects were children between one and seven years of age. After repeated injections, the children who had not had any HSV antibodies before the experiment (interpreted to mean that they had never had herpes) failed to develop any. The majority of subjects eventually contracted oral herpes, however, despite this attempt to prevent it.

In the early 1960s, the Eli Lilly research laboratories developed a formalin-inactivated preparation that was specific against HSV type-1, the type most often responsible for labial herpes. Even though initial studies in humans were not very encouraging (weekly injections over a ten-week period failed to stimulate antibody production), nonrandom placebo-controlled clinical trials were designed to determine whether injections of the preparations could diminish recurrences or lessen the severity of active infection.

In 1964 Drs. A. B. Kern and B. L. Schiff reported the results of their trials in the *Archives of Dermatology*. The preparation was not found to have any positive effect because test subjects who received the preparation experienced the same pattern of infection and the same rates of recurrence as subjects in the control group who were given a placebo. Lilly has since halted production of this preparation and no further human trials are anticipated.

By far the best-known specific immune stimulators are two preparations from Germany—Lupidon-G for genital herpes and Lupidon-H for oral herpes. Developed by a Hamburg firm, Hermal-Chemie, they utilize heat-inactivated viruses grown in embryonated chicken eggs. Therapy is complicated and consists of repeated injections at regular intervals over an extended period of time, often as long as a year. Unfortunately, the few results that have been reported provide no convincing support for claims of effectiveness.

In the March 1975 issue of *Skin Allergy News,* Dr. Theodore Nasemann of Frankfurt reported only marginal benefits using Lupidon-G in open trials. Recurrences were not prevented, and improvement of any kind was noted in only about half the subjects. Lacking any proof of efficacy, Lupidon-G and Lupidon-H have never been licensed for use in the United States, and the government of West Germany has recently suspended its use there.

At present, medical researchers have turned away from herpes simplex virus-specific immune stimulators because, after over forty years of experimentation, they have not been proven effective. There is little hope that such preparations have any place in the treatment of herpes.

Nonspecific Immune Stimulators

Even though the term *nonspecific immune stimulator* seems to defy what we know about the precise and quite specific way the body fights disease, the apparent contradiction is easily explained, at least theoretically, by the overall performance of the immune system.

The end products of the immune process—antibodies, killer cells, macrophages, and lymphoblasts—may be deficient in their disease-destroying potential for any number of reasons. The amount of antibody produced may be substandard because plasma cells are defective, insufficient in number, or simply poor producers of antibody. The function of killer cells may be inadequate because they are not overly receptive to the germ markers (antigens) that stimulate the hunt or because the poison they produce, lymphotoxin, isn't sufficiently lethal. The eating and digesting power of macrophages may be hampered because they lack the sensitivity to rush to the scene of infection in large numbers, because their digestive enzymes aren't up to par, or because they take one gulp and move away too quickly. And, finally, the action of lymphoblasts may be less than completely effective because the lymphokines they produce may be weak.

If any of these defense components cannot perform adequately, the immune system will not provide complete protection. Sometimes these deficiencies are so subtle that they can't be measured and show up only when the body is challenged by a particularly persistent microbe, like herpes, or by a microbe the body has to fight unassisted by antimicrobial drugs, again like herpes.

The theory behind nonspecific immune stimulators is that by increasing the defensive potential of the immune system all members of the defense, when challenged, will perform their specific tasks aggressively, with dispatch, and with uniform adequacy.

Over the past decade almost every theoretically probable and conceivable nonspecific immune stimulator has been tested for effectiveness and safety in controlling herpes, including active smallpox vaccine, inactive smallpox vaccine, live oral polio vaccine, BCG (tuberculosis) vaccine, and influenza virus vaccine. Let's take a look at two—BCG and influenza virus vaccine—that are fairly representative of the scientific experimentation with this technique.

Bacillus Calmette-Guerin (BCG). BCG is a live-bacteria vaccine formulated to protect against tuberculosis, and is made from the bacterium that caused tuberculosis almost fifty years ago. After decades of culturing it in their laboratory, French immunologists Calmette and Guerin (after whom the vaccine is named) observed that the germ had changed in that although it no longer had the ability to cause an active case of tuberculosis it was still sufficiently like its former self to provoke an immune response when injected. Today BCG is used worldwide as a tuberculosis vaccine.

The idea of using BCG as a possible treatment agent for herpes was a direct outgrowth of cancer and immunologic research into the nature of the mechanisms involved in immune-system surveillance of its enemies. In the 1960s, cancer investigators began to experiment with a variety of substances and biologic preparations that, when given to patients, were thought to enhance the defensive potential of the immune system. (If you will recall, cancer involves not only cell irregularities but also a failure of the immune system to fight back.) BCG was one of the preparations tested.

The researchers found that laboratory mice immunized

with BCG were better able to fight artificially induced cancers than animal subjects that were not given BCG. The results were encouraging but, unfortunately, a problem was noted. The fact that only about half the mice given BCG could fight the cancer was not noteworthy, as none of the control animals could, either. The real problem was that the cancer actually grew faster in about 10 percent of the BCG-vaccinated mice than it did in the control mice. Researchers continued testing BCG, however, for it appeared evident that some form of immune-system stimulation was taking place. Trials conducted with a wider variety of lab animals—rats, hamsters, and guinea pigs—confirmed that BCG heightened the immune function in about half the recipients. This was encouraging even though the response wasn't uniform.

Scientists began looking for other evidence to support the hypothesis that BCG stimulated immune activity, particularly in humans. Luckily, such evidence was uncovered. Researchers studying medical records in Quebec—where governmental policy requires that children be immunized not only against the usual spectrum of such vaccine-preventable diseases as diphtheria, whooping cough, smallpox, measles, polio, rubella, and tetanus but also (using BCG) against tuberculosis—discovered that BCG-immunized children in Quebec seemed to be less affected by childhood leukemia than children who did not receive the BCG vaccination. On the basis of these findings, scientists began to incorporate BCG experimentally into the treatment of various forms of cancer; although the results have been mixed, they have been sufficiently encouraging to merit further work because it is clear that BCG does heighten immune response in some patients.

Encouraged by the finding that BCG is a nonspecific immune stimulator, herpes researchers, who had long sought a way to gear up the immune system, began to experiment with it as a potential treatment. The earliest experiments were conducted in 1972 by a team headed by Dr. Carl L. Larson at the University of Montana. Rabbits were immunized with BCG and then infected with herpes in their eyes. This method of introducing the virus always blinds the subjects, and in unimmunized rabbits it usually leads to encephalitis and death. In this study, however, the investigators reported that death was prevented, something of an achievement.

The following year, Dr. Larson's team conducted studies in mice. This time, the results weren't as encouraging. Dr. Larson reported that BCG alone failed to protect previously immunized female mice against the intravaginal introduction of HSV-2, although when it was used in combination with herpes antibodies some degree of protection was obtained.

The observation that BCG couldn't prevent infection led Dr. Larson and his team to investigate its usefulness among patients who already had herpes. Could BCG limit recurrences or make them less severe? In June 1974, they reported the results of an open trial using BCG with fifteen patients suffering from recurrent genital herpes. Twelve of these patients—a whopping 80 percent—were reported to have improved significantly, and eight of the twelve reported a complete cessation of recurrences. The problem with this impressive result is that, since it was tested in an open trial without controls, we don't know whether BCG was the operative factor or not.

In 1976, Dr. Stanley M. Bierman of the UCLA Center for Health Services reported the results of another open trial using BCG with thirty-eight patients clinically diagnosed as having severe recurrent genital herpes. Over a follow-up period of one year, eight of the patients remained free of recurrences, but the overwhelming majority—thirty—continued to get them, although sixteen persons felt that their recurrences were less severe. As before, the meaning of these uncontrolled results isn't clear. In his report on this study, however, Dr. Bierman summarized the results of another BCG study he had conducted in which controls were employed. Those findings demonstrated no lessening of recurrences, and only marginal improvement in lesion severity, among patients who had received BCG as compared to those who had received a placebo.

That same year, the results of a properly controlled clinical trial of BCG were reported by Dr. Lawrence Corey of the

University of Washington School of Medicine in Seattle. The test, which included over a hundred patients with recurrent genital herpes diagnosed by tissue culture, failed to demonstrate any differences in recurrence rates, duration of active infection, or lesion severity between the BCG group and the control group.

Based on the definitive nature of the study design, Dr. Corey's results are regarded by most herpes researchers as conclusive, and BCG is no longer being considered as a potentially useful agent in the treatment of herpes.

Influenza Virus Vaccine (IVV). In May 1979, Dr. Joseph B. Miller of the University of Alabama Medical Center reported the results of a ten-year open trial using an influenza virus vaccine (IVV) to treat forty-four patients suffering with genital or labial herpes. These findings, originally published in *Annals of Allergy,* were picked up by the general press and received wide attention throughout the world as a breakthrough treatment and possibly even a cure. On the basis of the little information available, such grandiose claims were completely unwarranted. Although IVV may yet be tested more extensively and may even be found to offer some benefit, Dr. Miller's study is all that now exists, and, as we will see, his data were hardly definitive.

According to Dr. Miller, the impetus to use IVV to treat herpes patients came from his and other allergists' observations that many patients with labial and genital herpes seemed to respond to injections with IVV. Lesions healed rapidly and recurrences could be aborted by injections at the first prodromal warning. Starting in 1969, Dr. Miller began to enroll his herpes patients as subjects in a test of IVV. The study group was completely open, consisting of the first forty-four patients he encountered, and there were no placebo controls or double-blind procedures.

While the results are encouraging, even miraculous, their impact was compromised by the use of an open-study design. Every patient was said to improve with IVV therapy; an impressive 92 percent of the subjects reported recurrences of shorter duration, and 84 percent reported fewer recurrences. Without controls, however, there is no way of telling what these numbers really mean.

Even so, if IVV is relatively safe why not go ahead and use it? It is true that IVV is considered safe when used as it was originally intended to be used—infrequently (once a year, often less)—for flu protection, but consider Dr. Miller's treatment schedule:

> The usual schedule of IVV treatment injections is on the basis of need, i.e., the injections are administered only when symptoms recur. Needs vary but in moderate attacks of herpes labialis usually two or three injections are required the first day, one or two the second day and one daily for another few days. In more severe attacks, they may be given three or four times each 24 hours without waiting for pain to recur. In rare cases of unusually persistent and recurrent genital lesions and zoster, injections may continue to be needed one or more times daily for weeks or months to maintain relief or to cause subsequent recurrence to become milder, briefer, and less frequent.

That is a lot of flu vaccine to be injecting people with, far more than most of us will get over an entire lifetime, and it is not known whether it is safe in such amounts. In fact, if IVV weren't already licensed for use against flu and therefore available to any doctor, the FDA would never approve it for general use in treating herpes on the basis of these inconclusive open-trial results.

DIETARY AGENTS

There is no question that how well we eat has some bearing on the proper functioning of our bodies and particularly on our ability to resist disease and fight infection. A certain complement of caloric intake and nutrients is required to furnish the cells, tissues, and systems in our bodies with the various fuels and raw materials needed for metabolic processes.

We know that nutritional imbalances, deficiencies, and excesses can lead directly to disease or dysfunction. Not enough iron can cause anemia; too much mercury can poison us. We also know that even if they are not a direct cause of disease, nutritional deficiencies can hamper antibody formation and macrophage activity and, in general, diminish the capacity of the immune system to fight back. Indirectly, these problems can lead to lowered resistance, thereby increasing the risk of infection or exacerbating a current illness because the raw materials needed by the body to mount an adequate defense simply aren't available.

The appreciation that nutritional status is a factor in natural resistance to disease, coupled with the frustration felt by both doctors and patients in trying to manage recurrent herpes without the benefit of a proven and effective treatment agent, has led to the suggestion of a number of dietary agents as potential treatments for herpes. The list is large and includes calcium, vitamin B-complex, lactobacillus acidophilus (a "good" bacterium found in yogurt and normally present in the large intestine of most people), seaweed, camomile tea, vitamin C, dietary zinc, and lysine. Three of these suggested dietary approaches—vitamin C, zinc (a mineral), and lysine/arginine (amino acids)—have been widely publicized in recent years.

Vitamin C (Ascorbate)

No dietary agent used in the treatment of herpes and other diseases has received more attention or sparked greater controversy than vitamin C, an essential nutritional element that can't be stored by the body and therefore needs to be replaced continually. We now acknowledge that a vitamin C deficiency can lead to a disease called scurvy, but the notion that vitamin C plays an important—perhaps all-important—role in host resistance and the immune system's ability to fight disease is not so widely acknowledged. It has had a wild and stormy history.

In the early 1900s, long before the advent of antibiotics, people employed a wide range of home remedies to treat illnesses and promote health, including roots, teas, herbs, elixirs, and tonics. After the influenza epidemic of 1918,

Frederick R. Klenner, then a young boy, observed that certain people who had eaten an herbal folk medicine seemed to have been untouched by this illness that claimed the lives of 20 million people. Apparently this made a strong and lasting impression on him, for almost twenty years later, Klenner, then a medical student, analyzed the herbal preparation and found it to contain high concentrations of the new substance, vitamin C, which had been identified by Albert Szent-Gyorgyi in 1932. Klenner believed that it was the vitamin C in the herb that had made the crucial difference. His postulate was not altogether unreasonable in light of another recent discovery—that human beings were among only a handful of animals that couldn't manufacture their own vitamin C.

Throughout the late 1930s and 1940s, Dr. Klenner and many other physicians began to employ vitamin C clinically, as a therapeutic agent in the treatment of a wide variety of human illnesses. And, as had always been the practice, these physicians recorded their impressions and case experiences and reported them in medical and scientific journals. The reports were nothing short of fantastic.

High oral dosages and intravenous injections of vitamin C were said to cure polio, viral encephalitis, pneumonia, mononucleosis, rabies, influenza, and colds. Vitamin C therapy was also said to neutralize snake-bite poisoning and promote rapid healing following surgery. Furthermore, all of this was accomplished without any injurious side effects. Vitamin C was certainly beginning to look like the panacea for which humanity had been searching. Or was it?

In terms of traditional scientific rigors, the "evidence" of vitamin C's effectiveness wasn't evidence at all. The case reports and claims represented little more than clinical impressions and subjective observations made by well-meaning practitioners without any regard for proper experimental design or appropriate controls. And, frankly, unsubstantiated as these miraculous claims were, belief in them represented a leap of faith and little else, a leap most physicians found impossible to make.

There remained, however, a nucleus of doctors, chemists, and many lay people who continued to believe in the curative potential of large dosages of vitamin C, although they clearly weren't part of the mainstream of medicine, which acknowledged the nutritional importance of vitamin C, but in amounts far lower than advocated by its boosters.

From time to time, professional and public interest in vitamin C was rekindled as reports appeared in medical journals and lay publications. In a 1949 issue of the *British Journal of Nutrition,* G. H. Bourne, a British scientist, presented a comprehensive review of vitamin C and its relation to immunity, suggesting that human beings might require greater amounts of the substance than appeared to be necessary for dietary sufficiency alone.

The next year, Dr. Klenner reported that large dosages of vitamin C could cure measles, and throughout the 1950s and 1960s reports from Japan, England, Poland, and the United States credited high dosages of the vitamin with curing high blood pressure, kidney disease, prostate infections, heart disease, obesity, tumors, mental illness, and even herpes. (The popular "cure" of the day for herpes was 7 to 10 grams of vitamin C daily—roughly a hundred times more than recommended allowances—and the application of vitamin C cream on the sores ten to fifteen times a day.) As always, the reports were little more than subjective observations of a few cases without any scientific validation, but, as always, public interest was aroused.

In 1970, vitamin C was catapulted into the spotlight of intense medical and public interest when Nobel Prize winner Dr. Linus Pauling published his controversial book, *Vitamin C and the Common Cold.* Dr. Pauling contended that vitamin C stimulated natural immune mechanisms that were particularly effective against viral diseases in general, and specifically effective against the common cold. He concluded that, to be protective, "optimum daily intake of vitamin C for most adult human beings lies in the range of 2.3 grams to 9 grams," some 50 to 200 times more than previously thought necessary. Although the book itself was not intended as a scientific endeavor, the mere fact that such a recognized and respected scientist as Dr. Pauling had written it produced a response from the scientific community.

Three researchers at the University of Toronto, Drs. T. Anderson, D. Reid, and G. Beaton, designed a double-blind placebo-controlled experiment to test Dr. Pauling's hypothesis. A study group consisting of 407 persons was given daily dosages of vitamin C ranging from 1 to 4 grams; a matched control group of 411 persons received placebos. After two months, no difference was noted in the incidence of colds suffered by either group.

This well-designed study should have laid the issue to rest, but it didn't. The "cold trials," as they came to be called, were criticized for failing both to employ high enough dosages and to take into account the presumed immunosuppressive effect of sugar (sugar was thought to counteract the beneficial effect of vitamin C), which at the time was consumed at the annual rate of 150 pounds per person. Far from being resolved, the debate was still very much alive, and for the majority of scientists the question of whether vitamin C could activate the immune system against viral infections remained unanswered. Further studies were not proposed or conducted, and throughout most of the 1970s the status of vitamin C reverted to what it had been twenty years earlier: a matter of belief.

In 1979, Gary B. Thurman and Allan Goldstein, biochemists at George Washington University in Washington, D.C., began controlled experiments on vitamin-C-deprived guinea pigs (which, like humans, don't manufacture their own vitamin C). Thurman and Goldstein documented for the first time that vitamin C does indeed play some role in triggering or increasing immune responses.

The researchers infected seventy-four guinea pigs with a bacterium and thereafter fed all the animals a diet lacking only vitamin C. Half the guinea pigs, however, received supplements of the vitamin in their water, at dosages somewhat higher than would have been provided by their normal diet. The health status of both groups of animals was closely monitored, and each week they underwent tests to determine their lymphocyte and antibody responses.

Three weeks into the experiment, tissue levels of vitamin C in the group not receiving supplements had declined to low concentrations; the other group remained stable. In addition, lymphocyte and antibody response became very depressed in the vitamin-C-deprived group, whereas immune response appeared normal in the others. Perhaps most revealing, however, was that more than twice as many of the deprived guinea pigs died. Thurman and Goldstein concluded that the immune system needs vitamin C to mount a defense against infection, at least a bacterial infection like tuberculosis.

Encouraged by these immediate results, they then went after and obtained additional evidence that vitamin C is needed for immune response. Those vitamin-C-deprived guinea pigs who hadn't already died were given daily supplements for four weeks. Within two weeks, their lymphocyte and antibody responses started to improve, and in the third and fourth weeks they began to recover from the infection.

The results of this well-designed study are clear, but their implications have yet to be sorted out. While Thurman and Goldstein conclusively proved that complete deprivation of vitamin C will hamper the proper functioning of a guinea pig's immune systems, the state of total vitamin C deprivation is in itself clearly artificial. Precisely how these results may apply to guinea pigs and, ultimately, people in a non-totally-deprived state is not yet known and will be the subject of further investigations by these scientists. They intend to do research on how much vitamin C is really needed and on whether either benefit or harm may result from elevated dosages.

Does vitamin C cure disease, and, specifically, does it cure herpes? It is doubtful that vitamin C cures anything except diseases caused by vitamin C deficiency. Some daily amount of the vitamin appears to be needed—perhaps the 45 to 60 milligrams recommended by the FDA or the 500 to 1,000 milligrams proposed by some researchers, including Thurman and Goldstein. As for the extremely high dosages recommended by vitamin C adherents, without scientific evidence to back them up all you can do is make the leap of faith and believe.

Dietary Zinc

Zinc has been recognized as an essential nutritional factor in animals and humans for fifty years. Since the original observation in the 1920s that zinc was a dietary necessity, numerous findings have confirmed its role in growth and reproduction and as an important component of several metabolic enzymes.

There is no dispute that zinc is an important trace element, but so are iron, copper, and manganese. How did the notion arise that zinc might have therapeutic value in cases of herpes? First, zinc is incorporated into cell membranes and may serve to reinforce them, which led to the conclusion that viruses and other invasive organisms might have more difficulty gaining access to cells reinforced by zinc. Indeed, zinc seems to concentrate naturally in wounded tissues and is often used as a supplement in cases of burns, wounds, and bone fractures. According to biochemist Dr. Richard Passwater, zinc may promote healing by strengthening a cell's integrity and making it more resistant to disease.

Second, experiments performed in vitro have demonstrated that zinc possesses antiviral properties. Dr. Patrick O. Tennican, a herpes researcher who has been exploring zinc at the Arizona Health Science Center, reported that minute concentrations of zinc in herpes cultures using human cells caused marked reduction of viral activity without harming uninvaded cells.

Finally, some investigators have speculated that zinc is either used up more quickly or eliminated by the body during periods of physical or mental stress, and that therefore more of it may be needed during these periods. Stress, remember, may be a factor in recurrences of herpes.

At some point (the details are unclear), it was concluded that increased amounts of dietary zinc might prove beneficial as a treatment for herpes. Reports of using zinc dietary supplements ranging from 30 to 120 milligrams per day (two to eight times the recommended daily allowance) to treat herpes began appearing in popular-health and other magazines. Although no improvement was noted in some of the cases, many were encouraging and cited decreased severity and less frequent attacks. Of course, they were mere testimonials, not studies.

In late 1978, while exploring the possible benefit of topical zinc in the treatment of herpes, Dr. Tennican conducted an experiment that had some bearing on the effect of dietary zinc. Laboratory mice were infected vaginally with herpes and then were divided into three groups. One group was treated topically with a preparation of zinc sulfate, another received no treatment, and yet another was treated internally with zinc. After two weeks, the group of mice receiving zinc sulfate topically fared best; there were fewer deaths (herpes can kill a mouse) and the disease was less severe than among the untreated mice.

Of more interest to us, however, is the finding that the groups of untreated and internally treated mice did equally poorly. Both groups were subject to far more death and disease severity than the group treated topically. Dr. Tennican offered two possible explanations for the failure of systemic (internally administered) zinc. He postulated that the zinc was unable to concentrate in vaginal tissues in sufficient strength and that systemic use of zinc might even have depressed the animals' immune responses in light of the fact that there were more deaths among the mice receiving zinc internally than in any other group.

Given the disappointing animal studies conducted by Dr. Tennican and the absence of any well-controlled human experiments, there is no evidence to support a therapeutic role for dietary zinc in the treatment of herpes. Uncontrolled reports of successes with dietary zinc may well be attributed to the placebo effect. One word of caution: According to Dr. Passwater and others, high levels of zinc can be toxic. In general, it would be impossible to consume a toxic dose in food, but zinc supplements used to excess can prove damaging. Check with a doctor if you are ever inclined to supplement your diet with zinc.

Lysine and Arginine

Over the past five years, a number of articles have appeared in medical journals, health-food magazines, and the general press reporting that lysine and arginine, two of the eight essential amino acids, could influence the frequency and severity of recurrent herpes. Greater concentrations of lysine in relation to arginine were said to suppress recurrences, and greater concentrations of arginine in relation to lysine were said to promote them. The reports indicated that recurrences could be controlled by lysine supplements and by restricting foods known to be rich in arginine.

Lysine and arginine are neither new drugs nor antiviral compounds but elements found in most people's diets. In the discussion of nutritional requirements for protein in Chapter 5, we learned that the body manufactures all but eight of the amino acids that make up proteins, and that these eight—the essential amino acids—must be supplied in our diets. Lysine, one of the eight, is found in milk, red meat, brewer's yeast, and potatoes. Arginine, another, is found in peanuts, chocolate, and raw cereals. These two natural amino acids are believed to play a role in the growth pattern of herpes simplex viruses.

Amino acids, the essential building blocks of life, are required by every cell in our bodies. The herpes simplex viruses, which invade cells and use cellular machinery and raw materials to duplicate, use these amino acids. In 1952, while seeking to determine the amino-acid requirements of encephalomyelitis viruses, a research team headed by a scientist named Pearson found that, in vitro, high concentrations of lysine seemed most effective in slowing the rate of viral growth. By adding lysine to a culture medium containing viruses, Pearson demonstrated that the number of new viruses manufactured could be cut dramatically.

In 1964, a herpesvirus research team headed by Dr. R. W. Tankersley at the University of Richmond discovered that it wasn't just lysine that suppressed the growth of herpesviruses in culture medium; it was the relative concentration of lysine in relation to arginine. Dr. Tankersley demonstrated that by increasing lysine and holding arginine constant, viral growth was inhibited. Likewise, by cutting back on arginine and holding lysine constant, the same result could be achieved. And by eliminating lysine entirely or by adding arginine so that its concentration was greater than that of lysine, he showed that viral growth could be enhanced.

Dr. Tankersley concluded that herpes simplex viruses preferred greater concentrations of arginine for growth; in 1970, Dr. A. S. Kaplan provided validation by demonstrating that formation of the herpes simplex virus required three times as much arginine as lysine and that lysine inhibited the utilization of arginine in the manufacture of new viruses in cells.

In 1974, Dr. Christopher Kagan of the UCLA School of Medicine noted the previous work on lysine and arginine in vitro and hypothesized that the inhibitory effect of elevated lysine and/or decreased arginine on viral reproduction might be clinically useful in treating patients with herpes. Dr. Kagan instituted a limited, uncontrolled human trial using dietary supplements to test his hypothesis. In January 1974, he reported the results of this preliminary probe in *The Lancet,* a medical journal: "L-lysine 390 mg. was given orally at the first indication of onset of herpetic oral lesions in eight patients and vulvar lesions in two patients, with uniform rapid resolution of the lesions. This suggests that physicians in a position to study the effect of lysine in H. simplex infections should do so. It appears to do no harm and may be a useful therapeutic measure."

Later that year, encouraged by his preliminary findings, Dr. Kagan enlisted the cooperation of Dr. Richard S. Griffith from Wishard Memorial Hospital and Dr. Arthur L. Norins from the Indiana University School of Medicine to initiate a broader test of orally administered lysine as a therapeutic approach to herpes. The study was designed as an open trial with no controls against the placebo effect or investigator bias, and evaluation was based on before-and-after differences in recurrence rates and duration of symptoms as reported by patients or observed by the investigators.

A total of forty-five patients who sought treatment for genital and labial herpes lesions were enrolled as subjects in this experiment—thirty-four women and eleven men. Only nine of the patients had tissue-culture-proven herpes; the others had been diagnosed clinically. Subjects were counseled to limit their intake of foods known to be rich in arginine (seeds, nuts, and chocolate) and to take dietary supplements of lysine in the amount of 312 to 500 milligrams daily when not experiencing a recurrence. During active infection, the daily lysine supplement was increased to between 800 and 1,000 milligrams. Although some subjects were followed for as long as three years, most were followed for six months or less.

In 1978, Drs. Kaplan, Griffith, and Norins published their findings in the medical journal *Dermatologica.* They reported that, compared with past experiences, most patients seemed to suffer fewer outbreaks, and the outbreaks were less intense and of a shorter duration. Two patients benefited only marginally and two others not at all. There were no instances of adverse reactions to lysine.

On the basis of this open trial, the investigators cautiously concluded that relatively low-dosage supplements of dietary lysine might be beneficial in controlling recurrent herpes. They suggested that lysine enrichment works in vivo, as in vitro, to inhibit the growth of the virus and, therefore, to suppress but not cure herpes. In apparent acknowledgment of the weakness of their study design, Kagan, Griffith, and Norins' report called for more elaborate controlled studies of lysine.

In late 1978, in an article in *The Lancet,* Danish scientists Drs. Nils Milman, Jens Scheibel, and Ove Jessen reported the results of their trials with lysine in the treatment of herpes labialis. Their experience was not favorable.

The Danes had designed a double-blind placebo-controlled experiment in which patients began taking daily dosages of 1,000 milligrams of dietary lysine at the earliest sign of a recurrence and maintained this dosage for five and a half days; the controls received capsules containing ordinary cornstarch. A total of 104 patients participated (fifty-three received lysine and fifty-one received a placebo), and the study took nearly a year to complete.

The final tabulations demonstrated that recurrence rates, lesion severity, and healing patterns did not differ between the two groups. The general disappointment of the investigators was somewhat tempered, however, as they had not yet tried to prevent recurrences by using maintenance doses between episodes. They have begun to test lysine preventively, but results aren't in yet.

Can lysine be of some benefit in treating herpes? Probably not, at least as indicated by the definitive work of Milman, Scheibel, and Jessen. Can low-dosage dietary supplements of lysine taken daily suppress recurrences? Kagan's open-trial testing certainly points in that direction, but we will have to wait for more definitive studies.

TOPICAL AGENTS

Long before the development of modern scientific methods and advanced medical technology, and long before our understanding of the body and disease had progressed sufficiently to permit us to use these methods and technology, remedies and treatments were sought for the painful, distressing, and recurring lesions of herpes. Then, as now, the disease was troublesome enough to provoke a search for its solution.

The most common remedies and treatments had a basis in herbal medicine or folk practices and were usually topical preparations applied directly to the sores to relieve pain, itching, oozing, and discomfort. Boiled cloves and tea leaves, peppermint oil, clove oil, eucalyptus oil, pastes made from cornstarch, honey, slippery elm, comfrey root, myrrh, or volcanic ash, cactus sap, and milk compresses were among the many concoctions employed to relieve the symptoms of the disease. For the most part, these agents could be counted on to afford a measure of relief and comfort where otherwise there wasn't any, whether because of the placebo effect or actual pharmacologic activity. And, of course, in a relatively short time symptoms subsided and cleared up (as they do even if left alone), which served to reinforce the continued use of these "remedies."

In a sense, we have never stopped using these early medicinal substances. While eucalyptus oil or slippery-elm paste may not be prescribed today as a treatment for herpes, many agents in the modern therapeutic arsenal lack proven medicinal action and reflect the same basic motivation and philosophy of their predecessors: to give solace and support to the suffering patient. While it is true that some newer treatments, such as ether and dye-light therapy, have been suggested and tried because they were based on well-founded scientific theories or sound principles, others—including ice —have simply reflected the frustrated attempts of doctors and patients alike to find something—anything—that works in treating the disease.

Ether

An editorial entitled "The Misery of Recurrent Herpes: What to Do" appeared in the November 6, 1975, of the *New England Journal of Medicine*. Written by Dr. Albert B. Sabin, discoverer of the oral polio vaccine, it dealt with the use of topical ether in the management of herpes.

Dr. Sabin suggested that, in addition to soothing the pain and discomfort of herpes sores, the topical use of ether might interfere with viral replication in local tissues and limit the number of cells that harbor the latent virus, possibly reducing future recurrences. He cited a number of theoretical medical reports as well as one personal communication from Dr. J. S. Pasricha, an Indian physician who told of his clinical experience with ether and extolled its virtues in treating patients with herpes. Dr. Sabin also cited personal experience in the use ether, in which he had achieved gratifying results treating himself, members of his family, friends, and associates. In closing, Dr. Sabin called for carefully designed and controlled clinical trials of ether as a candidate treatment for herpes.

Following the appearance of Dr. Sabin's editorial, many

physicians took issue with his claims and expressed contrary opinions in print. The ensuing controversy smoldered for the next three years.

In late 1978, Dr. Lawrence Corey and his associates at the University of Washington School of Medicine provided some answers in a *New England Journal of Medicine* article entitled "Ineffectiveness of Topical Ether for the Treatment of Genital Herpes Simplex Virus Infection." The investigators described the results of a one-year controlled study of ether (described in Chapter 4) involving fifty-six patients. No differences in recurrence rates or lesion severity were noted between the group receiving ether and the control group, although the group receiving ether seemed to take *longer* to heal. Dr. Corey and his colleagues not only concluded that ether doesn't work but, because it burns when applied, he questioned ether's soothing effect as well.

Subsequent studies of ether at the University of Utah College of Medicine have confirmed Dr. Corey's findings. Ether is no longer regarded as a potentially useful treatment agent for herpes.

Ice Therapy

Ordinary ice was termed an "effective remedy" for herpes by Israeli physician Dr. Stanford Danziger in a letter published in *The Lancet* in which he reported achieving clinical success with fourteen herpes patients who used his recommended ice procedure.

Dr. Danziger's treatment method was the continuous application of ice cubes to the site of lesions for a period of an hour and a half to two hours. Upon initiation of this therapy, pain is said to subside immediately because the coldness numbs the area, and although feeling returns after the ice is removed, Dr. Danziger reports that the pain ceases entirely. The following day the lesions disappear and healing is complete within one or two days.

Dr. Danziger stressed that, to be effective, his therapy

must be started within twenty-four hours of the development of lesions and that, even when effective, prompt healing is the best result that can be achieved. Recurrences are not prevented by the application of ice. Two additional considerations were cited regarding this approach. First, topical use of ice is so harmless that it can be done at home. Second, there are difficulties in maintaining the ice cube in contact with sores for one and a half to two hours.

Based on Dr. Danziger's description of his treatment and the results he obtained among a limited number of patients, Dr. David R. Zimmerman, author of a medical column in *Ladies' Home Journal,* suggested that readers with herpes try the ice-cube technique and report their reactions by letter. The results of this informal poll were summarized in a letter from Dr. Zimmerman published by *The Lancet.* Over a period of four months, Dr. Zimmerman had received twenty-six letters from patients, twenty-five of whom said the method resulted in dramatic improvement; the other reported only slight benefit. Although the findings were obviously unconfirmed and informal, Dr. Zimmerman felt it significant that no one wrote to say that the ice method had been attempted without success.

Are the results significant? Might some benefit be derived from using the ice cube technique? No and maybe. No, the results cannot be termed significant in any scientific respect. The number of patients in Dr. Danziger's trial was very small, and no attempt was made to control against the placebo effect. Dr. Zimmerman's informal poll, in addition to sharing these two defects, also lacked any semblance of objectivity: twenty-six people furnished personal, subjective interpretations of their experiences with ice, and no one can be sure that their sores were even caused by the herpes simplex virus.

Maybe some sufferers would benefit by using the ice-cube technique. The extreme cold can certainly provide relief from the pain or soreness that may accompany herpes lesions. As for promoting rapid healing, however—who knows? The ice may have served as an inducement for the patient to want to get better rapidly.

Dye-Light Treatment

The concept that viruses can be inactivated if they are exposed to a combination of light and certain photoreactive dyes was originated in the early 1900s when an investigator observed that a certain light-reactive dye was harmless to a one-celled microbe in the dark but lethal to it in the presence of light. Early research on viruses demonstrated that they were light-sensitive as well, and in the 1960s herpes simplex viruses were found to be inactivated by exposure to both light and certain photoreactive dyes.

In 1972, a research team headed by the noted virologist and epidemiologist Dr. Joseph L. Melnick, of the Baylor College of Medicine in Houston, experimented with dye-light therapy on rabbits with herpes keratitis and noted encouraging results. Following this experiment, the procedure was attempted on human subjects with herpes simplex virus infections of the lips, skin surface, mouth, and genital areas. In the January 15, 1973, issue of the *Journal of the American Medical Association,* Dr. Melnick reported the treatment to be highly successful in that sores treated with dye-light healed more rapidly, and there were fewer recurrences than among the control group.

The activating mechanism of this technique, in which sores are painted with a photoreactive dye and then exposed to light of a particular wavelength and intensity, was presumed to involve the ability of the dye to fit into the genetic material of the virus and, upon exposure to light, to cause disruption and fragmentation of the viral genes, thereby preventing the virus from reproducing itself and infecting other cells. At this early juncture, the outlook for dye-light therapy certainly looked promising; however, a major controversy was about to begin.

In the July 30, 1973, issue of the *Journal of the American Medical Association,* Dr. Fred Rapp, a distinguished microbiologist at the Pennsylvania State University College of Medicine and a former associate of Dr. Melnick's, reported that photoinactivation treatment of herpes simplex infections represented a potentially dangerous procedure. He based his conclusions on laboratory experiments with animals which indicated that, although the dye-light procedure reduced the infectiousness of herpes simplex viruses, the fragments of the virus that remained were capable of transforming normal cells into cancer cells.

The debate next moved onto the pages of the February 22, 1974, issue of *Medical World News*, where Dr. Rapp reiterated his earlier caution and introduced a new one—that during the treatment process the dye might enter uninfected cells, fit into the DNA of such cells, and, upon exposure to light, cause fragmentation of normal cellular DNA along with any effect it might have on the virus. "In theory at least," he said, "you could convert a normal cell into a malignant cell without any interaction of a virus at all."

Dr. Melnick dismissed the danger of potential cell transformation by the virus, stating that increased light-exposure time led to more complete inactivation. He responded to the issue of possible damage to proximate uninfected cells by stating, "Only if we add a tremendous excess of dye to normal cells will the cells be damaged."

Dr. Rapp contended that this rebuttal had missed his point: "The hooker in photoinactivation is that defective viruses are often cancer viruses. We have evidence from this laboratory and from about eight other laboratories that rendering herpes simplex viruses defective still allows them to transform cells in vitro. To do that, a virus requires only a piece of its DNA, not the whole thing."

In the November 6, 1975, issue of the *New England Journal of Medicine*, Dr. Martin G. Myers and his team at Harvard Medical School reported the results of their placebo-controlled study of dye-light therapy in the treatment of herpes, a report that was to mark the beginning of the end for this procedure. Dr. Myers reported that dye-light treatment failed to make a difference in either healing patterns or recurrence rates among test subjects as compared with controls. The group at Harvard concluded that, in the absence of demonstrated effectiveness, the routine use of dye and light in patients with recurrent herpes should be discontinued.

Today dye-light treatment is no longer recommended as a procedure for managing herpes. In an interview conducted in late 1978, Dr. Rapp succinctly summarized the prevailing medical opinion: "Here is a treatment that is probably hazardous and also doesn't work. It should not be used by the practicing clinician."

AFTERTHOUGHTS

So there we have it—an array of would-be "cures," past and present, that seem to bear out this medical axiom: "If there are many proposals for therapy, no one must be good." Is this where it ends? Hardly. As a matter of fact, we've only just begun.

In a way, all the cures we have covered, and dozens of others, were necessary stopping-off points on the research-and-development road of medicine. True, most have resulted in failure, but from failure we get more answers, better questions, and a clearer sense of where *not* to look. This is precisely what has happened. Research to find an effective treatment and maybe even a cure for herpes is alive and well and bears no resemblance to the simplistic work of the past. For, as we will see in the next chapter, the day of antiviral chemotherapy is about to dawn.

CHAPTER 11

FUTUREHOPE: THE POSSIBILITY OF A CURE

One day in the future, herpes will no longer be the personal and public-health problem it is today. There will be vaccines to confer immunity against these viruses and fully curative and safe antiviral agents to eradicate the viruses among those already infected. It is difficult to predict when such scientific breakthroughs will occur, given the many complexities and problems that still remain unsolved, but in view of the research interest and effort in antiviral drug development during the past decade, it is inevitable that they will occur. In fact, some have already.

Ten years ago, doctors could do little about herpes keratitis except hope that the patient's own defenses were strong enough to overcome the virus and prevent blindness. Today we can cure it. Just five years ago, herpes encephalitis was usually fatal. Today antiviral drugs can save the patient.

The problems that must be overcome are many, and some are awesome, but today's molecular biologists, pharmacologists, virologists, and immunologists are well-matched opponents to a worthy viral challenger. To understand some of the complexities that face them, let's briefly review some of the material covered in this book.

In Chapter 3 we learned that herpes simplex viruses, like all viruses, are invasive intracellular parasites. Since they lack metabolic and reproductive self-sufficiency, they must enter a host cell and take it over to perpetuate themselves. This viral invasion of cells provokes natural immunologic defenses that limit the infection and ultimately cause herpes to lie dormant in nearby nerve cells.

In Chapter 4 we learned that this latent state is one of equilibrium between the host and the virus. As long as immune defenses remain sufficiently strong, the virus simply persists without replicating or causing cell destruction; but if resistance is lowered, the virus is able to reemerge as an active infection.

Unlike bacteria, which do not invade living cells and can be fought outside the cells, viruses must be attacked where they reside: inside the cells of our bodies. The ultimate objective of antiviral drug research, therefore, is to discover or formulate a substance that is (1) discriminating—able to distinguish between cells that are harboring the virus and those that are not; (2) selective—active against invaded cells without affecting normal cells; (3) potent—able to destroy the entire virus without leaving fragments that may cause later problems; and (4) nontoxic to the cell but lethal to the virus. The challenge imposed by these criteria is significant, so significant that just fifteen years ago few scientists believed it could be successfully met.

In 1965, the New York Academy of Sciences sponsored one of the first conferences on antiviral therapy. At that time there were fewer than six scientists in the United States who were confident that safe and effective antiviral substances could be developed. Most of the scientific community then believed that the replicative cycle of viruses was so like that of cells that it would be nearly impossible to find agents capable of interfering with the viral cycle without also killing normal cells.

In 1970, a second conference on antiviral chemotherapy was sponsored by the New York Academy of Sciences. In just five years the opinion of the scientific community had undergone a change. Investigators and researchers had begun to identify numerous differences between viral replication cycles and the reproductive activities of uninfected cells, and a large percentage of those present at the conference believed that these differences could be exploited.

In February 1976, the third conference on antiviral chemotherapy was attended by a community of believers. In fact, the age of antiviral agents had arrived. Most attention and discussion focused on several antiviral compounds that had been tested and found to be relatively safe and effective against a number of viral diseases, including herpes keratitis. The major questions for most conference participants related to when such agents could be marketed and how soon even better antiviral substances could be found. In little more than ten years, the medical world had done a complete about-face on the issue of antiviral chemotherapy.

One of the antiviral compounds discussed in 1976, and one of the first to reach the commercial market, was idoxuridine (IDU). This drug was the first agent found to be effective in preventing blindness in cases of herpes keratitis. Doctors also tried it for other forms of herpes, but when it was applied topically to sores IDU seemed to have no effect; when administered internally in an attempt to treat herpes encephalitis, IDU was found to interfere with the replicative cycle of normal cells to a dangerous extent and, therefore, was judged unsafe for systemic use. Despite its limited applicability, IDU was hailed by doctors and researchers as a breakthrough. It was a "first" in antiviral chemotherapy, comparable in importance to sulfa drugs and penicillin.

Research to find an antiviral drug safer than IDU continues, based on the differences between infected and uninfected cells. Early in 1979, the National Institute of Allergy and Infectious Diseases, one of the National Institutes of

Health, published the findings of a two-year Task Force on Viral Infections that drew upon the resources of the most prominent virologists, immunologists, and other related scientists in America today. Approximately one-fifth of its more than 1,000 pages was devoted to the control of viral infections. The following statement from the Task Force report summarizes one of the recommendations: "Virus multiplication consists of the synthesis of viral nucleic acids and proteins and their assembly into virus particles. A rational approach to antiviral chemotherapy should be to examine whether and where these processes can best be interrupted without interfering with the functioning of the host."

In somewhat greater detail, the report went on to define these differences:

1. In infected cells, replication of the genes of the herpes simplex viruses requires certain enzymes not normally formed in uninfected cells. Accordingly, "it should be possible to isolate and characterize these enzymes and to find or devise specific inhibitors for them." Replication of viral genes could be prevented and no new viruses would be produced.

2. The process by which infected cells manufacture viral parts appears to differ fundamentally from the process by which normal cells manufacture their own replacement parts. If a drug could recognize this fundamental difference and interfere with the process, cells would be prevented from building the necessary parts of a virus.

3. Once manufactured, the various parts of a virus are assembled into complete viruses within an infected cell. If the viral mechanisms that trigger this sequence can be indentified, drugs can be designed to prevent the assembly of complete viruses in cells.

The Task Force thus indentified three strategies for stopping viral infections: prevent viral genes from being manufactured, prevent other parts of the virus from being manufactured, and—in the absence of the ability to accomplish either of the preceding—prevent the assembly of the various viral parts into complete viruses.

Drugs whose action reflects any of the three strategies for inhibiting viral replication hold great promise as effective antiviral treatment agents. Such drugs probably won't be completely curative, however—at least not in the usual sense that we think of a cure. The action of antibiotics, for example, results in the elimination of every last bacterium from the body; subsequent infections after proper treatment are the result of new exposure. Antiviral drugs, on the other hand, work only during periods of active infection, when the viruses are actually replicating. While viruses are in their latent state, the drugs have no effect on them.

Despite this limitation, drugs that interrupt the cycle of viral replication are being researched and will be quite useful. By curbing the production of viruses, they can greatly curb the severity of acute infections, and by reducing the number of cells in which latent viruses can reside, they can reduce the chance of recurrences. The antiviral compounds that employ this strategy and are strong candidates as effective treatment agents for herpes include adenine arabinoside (ara-A), ribavirin, aciclovir (ACV), 2-Deoxy-d-glucose (DG), and phosphonoacetic acid (PAA).

Another approach to antiviral chemotherapy identified by the Task Force is to prevent viruses from invading new cells. As we have seen in Chapter 3, this is precisely what interferon does. Interferon, you will recall, is the chemical produced by infected cells and excreted for the benefit of uninfected neighboring cells, making them more resistant to viral invasion. Research scientists are pursuing interferon as an antiviral treatment agent in two ways: by trying to manufacture and purify it in large quantities in a laboratory for subsequent internal administration and by trying to develop drugs that will boost the body's ability to manufacture interferon naturally. We will examine interferon in detail later in this chapter but, first, let's evaluate those compounds that reflect the Task Force report's finding on viral replication.

VIRAL REPLICATION INHIBITORS
Adenine Arabinoside (ara-A)

Adenine arabinoside, commonly called ara-A, was first discovered to possess antiviral properties in 1964. French scientists were engaged in a massive screening effort to test samples of plant and animal substances from both land and sea in an effort to find possible anticancer agents. Ara-A, which comes from a Caribbean sponge, was among the substances tested. The scientists found that although ara-A did little to retard the growth of cancer cells, it did interfere with viral activity.

Results from early tests of ara-A in vitro confirmed that ara-A inhibited the synthesis of viral genes. Only three potential problems were noted, none of which precluded the development and subsequent use of ara-A.

The first problem was that ara-A was found to be teratogenic—that is, it could cause birth defects. This finding did not come as a surprise, and was in fact anticipated. Teratogenicity seems to be a characteristic of many of the antiviral compounds that work by inhibiting viral gene synthesis, because the enzymes involved in the rapid cell division that takes place during gestation may be similar to viral enzymes in infected cells. The danger of birth defects, however, can be eliminated by avoiding the drug's use in pregnant women.

The second problem—the insolubility of ara-A in water—made administration of the drug more difficult. Ara-A has to be given intravenously in relatively small amounts over a longer period. If it were water-soluble, ara-A could be injected with little difficulty.

The third and most troublesome problem was the finding that ara-A was rapidly decomposed by a naturally occurring enzyme in humans called adenine deaminase. Decomposition of ara-A resulted in an altered form of the drug that is somewhat less active. Overcoming this problem required higher doses of ara-A or the use of ara-A in combination with a specific inhibitor of the enzyme adenine deaminase. The latter approach is less desirable because physicians prefer not to inhibit an enzyme that occurs naturally in the body.

Controlled in vivo testing of ara-A against several types of herpes infections yielded mixed results. On the plus side, ara-A was found to be quite effective against herpes keratitis. In studies conducted separately by Dr. Peter Laibson at the Wills Eye Hospital in Philadelphia and Dr. Deborah Pavan-Langston at the Massachussetts Eye and Ear Infirmary in Boston, ara-A was demonstrated to be at least as effective as idoxuridine, and it produced fewer side effects. It was further shown that ara-A could succeed in cases where idoxuridine failed or where the patient couldn't tolerate IDU.

As we saw in Chapter 9, controlled human trials of ara-A in the treatment of herpes encephalitis also proved highly successful. Drs. Charles A. Alford and Richard J. Whitely, at the University of Alabama, leading a team of over twenty investigators at fifteen universities in a four-year collaborative evaluation of the substance, reported their findings in the August 11, 1977, issue of the *New England Journal of Medicine.* They demonstrated that, if administered early enough in the course of the disease, ara-A will not only prevent death but will also radically reduce the incidence of brain damage in survivors.

Unfortunately, the positive effects of ara-A in relation to herpes keratitis and encephalitis could not be demonstrated in treating surface lesions among victims of recurrent herpes. In 1975, Dr. James P. Luby of the South Western Medical Center in Dallas reported the results of a placebo-controlled evaluation of topical ara-A in the treatment of genital herpes among men. The substance was found to be ineffective; no differences in rates of recurrence or healing were noted between the men receiving ara-A and the controls. Subsequent studies by Dr. King K. Holmes of the University of Washington School of Medicine and Dr. Spotswood L. Spruance of the University of Utah College of Medicine failed to demonstrate any effectiveness of ara-A among women with genital herpes or among any patients with labial herpes.

While, at the time of these studies, investigators could only speculate as to the reason for ara-A's ineffectiveness against genital and labial herpes, the prevailing opinion was that ara-A couldn't penetrate the skin and reach infected cells in sufficient concentrations to inhibit viral replication. This is now known to be true and a new technique called *iontophoresis* is being employed to enhance tissue penetration by ara-A. Iontophoresis involves the use of low concentrations of electrical current on the surface of the skin to drive the ara-A molecules into cells. This procedure has already been found to be effective in animal experiments, and human trials should be taking place soon.

Despite its present limitations, ara-A has proven to be a safe and effective agent against at least two of the more serious forms of herpes. It has been licensed by the FDA for internal use in the treatment of herpes encephalitis and for external use in the treatment of ocular herpes, and is commercially available as a prescription medicine under the trade name Vira-A.

Ribavirin

Ribavirin is similar to ara-A in that its antiviral properties also work by interfering with the synthesis of viral genes. The mechanism by which this occurs, however, is different, as is the fact that, unlike ara-A, which is a naturally occurring substance, ribavirin is commercially manufactured.

Ribavirin was synthesized in the laboratories of ICN Pharmaceuticals, Inc., of Irvine, California. According to scientists at ICN, ribavirin is designed to inhibit an enzyme— inosine monophosphate dehydrogenase—that enhances the biosynthesis of viral genetic information in cells infected by herpes simplex viruses (and by several other viruses as well; the action of ribavirin is fairly broad).

Studies of ribavirin's action in vitro have demonstrated it to be as effective as idoxuridine and ara-A against herpes simplex viruses, and experiments with animals have supported this finding. Human clinical trials with the drug were conducted in Mexico among patients suffering with herpes zoster, a disease in adults caused by reactivation of latent chickenpox viruses (varicella-zoster viruses, which are closely related to herpes simplex viruses). The experimental design was controlled for the placebo effect, and the results were encouraging. Topical application of ribavirin reduced the pain and severity of the sores (they appear around the midsection or back and follow the nerve pathways lying beneath the skin) and shortened the active course of the disease (like herpes simplex, herpes zoster has active and latent phases). In addition, very few side effects were noted.

Ribavirin has won approval for widespread use in Mexico, Brazil, and a number of other countries in Central and South America and Africa, where it is sold under the name Virazole. The FDA has not licensed it for sale in the United States pending the outcome of additional clinical trials.

Aciclovir (ACV)

In 1978, a North Carolina pharmaceutical company, Burroughs Wellcome Laboratories, announced that it had succeeded in developing a new antiviral compound known as aciclovir (ACV) that showed promise as a potential chemotherapeutic agent in the treatment of three herpesvirus infections: herpes simplex, herpes zoster, and infectious mononucleosis (caused by the Epstein-Barr herpes virus).

According to Burroughs Wellcome research director Dr. Gertrude Elion, aciclovir was discovered by a team of investigators headed by Dr. Howard Schaeffer. In the course of conducting complex experiments to alter the molecular structure of crystalline compounds known as purines and test their antiviral potential, Dr. Schaeffer's team found that one of the altered compounds—BW248U (now called aciclovir, or ACV)—to be the most active agent yet observed against herpes growth in cell cultures. They measured its potency as a hundred times greater than that of ara-A.

The scientists sought to determine the reason for aciclovir's high antiviral activity against herpes-infected cells and found that the drug closely resembled the enzyme thymidine kinase, a substance used in the replication of the herpes simplex virus. In the process of replicating, the virus will erroneously use ACV to build new genetic material. Since ACV is not identical but only similar to the necessary substance, the virus' genes are incomplete, and it is destroyed. In the words of Dr. Elion, "The virus commits suicide."

Burroughs Wellcome scientists discovered another major advantage of ACV: its highly selective action against herpes-infected cells and its "ignorance" of uninfected cells. The enzyme thymidine kinase is found only in herpes-infected cells, so only infected cells will mistakenly seize upon the drug for use in viral replication. According to Harvard ophthalmologist Dr. Deborah Pavan-Langston, who will be testing ACV in cases of herpes keratitis: "What makes ACV unique is that it is activated only by cells containing the herpesvirus and thereby spares normal cells. As a result, it is both potent and safe."

Early studies in animals have shown that aciclovir can be given orally without alteration by the digestive system and that the concentrations of the drug reaching the bloodstream are sufficient for antiviral activity. In addition, Burroughs Wellcome scientists have demonstrated that ACV can be given intravenously to rats, guinea pigs, rabbits, and mice in order to achieve even higher blood concentrations without becoming toxic.

On the basis of these very encouraging early results, three applications for experimentation with ACV in humans have been approved by the FDA: its use as an ointment to be applied in the eyes for the treatment of herpes keratitis; its use intravenously for the treatment of systemic herpes in babies and herpes encephalitis in adults; and its use as a topical ointment for treating oral and genital herpes. Very carefully designed controlled experiments are in progress at this time. Preliminary results will not be available until late 1980 or early 1981, but optimism and excitement about the drug are high.

Assuming that the results of these limited trials are as encouraging as the earlier animal work, ACV will be ready to receive widespread testing. The testers will need to develop dosage levels and treatment schedules as well as define various parameters relating to possible toxicity, metabolic activity, and blood levels. If ACV is found to be as safe and effective as it appears to be, it will make a major difference in our ability to treat herpes.

2-Deoxy-d-glucose (DG)

In the June 29, 1979, issue of the *Journal of the American Medical Association,* Drs. Herbert A. Blough and Robert L. Giuntoli from the University of Pennsylvania School of Medicine reported the results of a two-year placebo-controlled limited human trial of a substance called 2-Deoxy-d-glucose (DG) in the treatment of genital herpes. Their report was entitled "Successful Treatment of Human Genital Herpes Infections with 2-Deoxy-d-glucose," and, as the title implies, the substance looks very promising.

Although its present form and use as an antiviral chemotherapeutic agent in the treatment of genital herpes are new, 2-Deoxy-d-glucose has been known for some time. In 1959, Dr. Edwin D. Kilbourne, presently head of microbiology at the Mount Sinai School of Medicine in New York, suggested that DG might be an effective antiviral compound. Dr. Kilbourne was attracted to the drug because of its relatively low toxicity, but studies with it were abandoned when he found that it had no effect on influenza virus in mice under laboratory conditions. Thus the potential antiviral properties of DG remained essentially unexplored for the next fourteen years.

In the medical journal *Virology* in 1973, a research team that included Dr. Blough reported that 2-Deoxy-d-glucose was capable of interfering with the viral-mediated function of fusion, one of the methods in which herpes simplex viruses spread from cell to cell without being exposed to potentially lethal extracellular chemicals. Just a year later, other investigators found that the substance was capable of interfering with the replication of herpes simplex viruses, and less than a year after that, a report appeared in *Virology* addressing the question of how 2-Deoxy-d-glucose acts on virus-infected cells. It was found that, unlike ara-A, ribavirin, and aciclovir, which interfere with the synthesis of viral genetic material, DG acts to inhibit the assembly of complete viral particles; in other words, it blocks the formation of the envelope that surrounds herpes simplex viruses—and without an envelope, the virus is destroyed.

With a reasonable understanding of how and why 2-Deoxy-d-glucose derives its antiviral properties, in 1977 Drs. Blough and Giuntoli initiated a well-controlled human clinical trial of the agent among fifty-one women with either primary or recurrent genital herpes. Every case had been diagnosed by tissue culture except one, which had been confirmed using other laboratory techniques. The women were divided into two groups: a treatment group of thirty-six and a placebo group of fifteen. After the initial treatment and evaluations, recurrence patterns were monitored for a two-year follow-up period. The results of the trial were quite interesting and very encouraging.

Among women experiencing their first episode of genital herpes, those who received the test drug (DG) took less than half the time to heal as those who received the placebo. During the two-year follow-up period, only 11 percent of those who were treated experienced a recurrence, as opposed to 35 percent among the controls. Among women with recurrent herpes, those receiving the drug healed in approximately half the time as those in the placebo group. During the two-year follow-up period, every woman who had received placebos experienced at least one recurrent attack, but only 45 percent of the women treated with the experimental drug developed recurrences.

These findings suggest that 2-Deoxy-d-glucose might serve as an effective chemotherapeutic agent in controlling genital herpes among women. Safety does not appear to be an issue, as no toxic side effects were noted. In the hope that these preliminary successes can be extended to men, and to both men and women with other forms of herpes, studies are under way to test the drug's effectiveness among men, in cases of herpes keratitis and herpes encephalitis, and among immunosuppressed herpes patients of both sexes.

At present, the drug is strictly limited to an experimental

substance by the FDA. If these favorable preliminary findings are borne out by further testing in Philadelphia and at other clinical centers, 2-Deoxy-d-glucose will become a candidate for widespread use by physicians in treating herpes.

Phosphonoacetic Acid (PAA)

Phosphonoacetic acid is a new antiviral agent being studied by researchers Lacy R. Overley and associates at the Abbott Laboratories in Chicago. PAA may well turn out to be one of the most effective antiherpes drugs yet discovered; it is certainly the most specific, as it acts only against herpesviruses.

Although it is the least tested of all the new antivirals, PAA has already been shown to have one theoretic advantage over ara-A, ribavirin, and aciclovir. Since it works to inhibit viral replication in a fundamentally different way than do these other three, PAA may not be as likely to cause birth defects. If this advantage is confirmed in testing, it may be possible to use PAA in cases where ara-A, ribavirin, and ACV are not indicated.

Thus far, PAA has been tried only on animals, but results appear to be encouraging. In tests conducted in 1977, it was found to be highly active in herpes-infected mice, more so than either IDU or ara-A. Furthermore, this high state of antiviral activity diminished less rapidly after treatment than did the activity of the other drugs.

Plans to move PAA out of the animal-testing phase and into human trials are impeded by the facts that PAA is not patentable as are ribarivin, aciclovir, and DG (pending) and that its action—and, therefore, its market—is limited only to herpesviruses. Whether or not Abbott Laboratories or some other pharmaceutical firm is willing, without patent protection, to invest the estimated $2.5 to $5 million in further development of PAA and human trials remains to be seen. There is precedent and hope, however, since the development of ara-A, which is also unpatentable, was energetically supported and financed by the pharmaceutical firm of Parke-Davis and Company. They have demonstrated that while patent protection against another firm's encroachment of an expensive development is important, an effective treatment agent for herpes—even one that could be manufactured by any drug company—can be commercially worth the investment as well as a boon to humanity.

INTERFERON: THE VIRAL INVASION REGISTER

Since the discovery in 1957 by Drs. Alick Isaacs and Jean Lindenmann that the body produces an antiviral substance of its own, interferon has been researched and investigated extensively for its action against viral infections, which possibly is analogous to the action of antibiotics against bacterial disease. Why all the interest in the chemical? Paraphrasing the NIAID Task Force report on viral infections, three properties place interferon at the forefront of potentially useful agents in the control of viral infections: (1) extremely high specific antiviral activity, (2) broad spectrum application (interferon works against all viruses), and (3) low toxicity. Interferon is unique in its ability to selectively inhibit the replication of a wide variety of viruses without necessarily affecting normal cellular functions. In short, interferon has provoked great scientific curiosity because it represents an ideal antiviral agent—highly active against viruses without being very toxic.

Unfortunately, interferon is also one of the most expensive substances in the world; to produce just one ounce would cost $100 million. Under natural circumstances, the cells of the body manufacture trace quantities of interferon, but far greater amounts are needed for research and clinical testing purposes. Toward this end, a Finnish scientist, Dr. Kari Cantell, has developed a method to produce interferon in a laboratory. He starts with large numbers of human leukocytes (white blood cells), which are derived by separating whole blood withdrawn for transfusion. He then challenges them with a viral agent, which causes them to produce interferon —human leukocyte interferon.

Retrieving the minuscule amounts of human leukocyte

interferon is the most difficult and expensive part of the procedure. The batch of biologic material contains leukocytes, viruses, nutrients to keep the leukocytes alive, and other fluids produced by the leukocytes along with a small quantity of interferon floating about. Dr. Cantell's process for extracting and purifying the interferon—a crucial step—is exceedingly formidable and expensive because gallons of white blood cells yield only drops of interferon pure enough for human use and research purposes. But, fortunately, we don't need much. Because of its high level of antiviral activity, interferon dosages for treatment and testing are measured in picograms—trillionths of a fluid ounce.

Perhaps because of its fantastic cost or because scientists have not yet determined its action and dosage levels, human leukocyte interferon has not yet been used extensively in clinical trials. In those few instances where it has been tested, results were encouraging. A particularly nasty condition of viral warts in the throats of children was treated somewhat successfully with interferon. The warts disappeared and then grew back (as they sometimes do), but they continued to respond to each successive interferon treatment. According to Dr. Hans Strandler, the interferon researcher who treated the children, "Repeated courses of interferon are infinitely easier on a child than repeated surgery." And at the Stanford University Medical Center, Dr. Thomas C. Merigan, another interferon researcher, has found the substance to be of value in treating herpes zoster in cancer patients whose weakened immune systems were unable to control the infection.

The experiments of Strandler and Merigan were limited, however, as both were open trials. Recently a team headed by Dr. G. J. Pazin at the University of Pittsburgh School of Medicine designed a placebo-controlled test of great interest to us, for the disease against which it was used was herpes labialis.

Surgery on the trigeminal sensory root (the nerve cluster in the cheek where the latent virus hides out) to relieve trigeminal neuralgia has been found to stimulate recurrences of labial herpes. Dr. Pazin and his team investigated the preventive potential of human leukocyte interferon in postsurgical reactivation of herpes. Thirty-seven patients were enrolled in the study, all of them similar in terms of age, sex, and frequency and severity of prior herpes lesions. All underwent the identical surgical procedure and received the same postoperative care and treatment. The only difference was that nineteen of them received roughly 5 million units of interferon (less than one drop) each day for five days, while the other eighteen received a placebo.

Following surgery, the overall recurrence rate in the placebo group was 83 percent. Among those who received interferon, the recurrence rate was 47 percent, and no adverse reactions were observed. Even though interferon failed to prevent recurrences in every member of the test group, the disparity in recurrence rates between the two groups is considered significant and serves to encourage further scientific experimentation with the substance.

Interferon Inducers

External production and purification is only one avenue of interferon research being pursued today. The great difficulties and cost of this process have naturally led investigators to examine the other way of producing interferon: in the body. Dr. Hilton B. Levy, of the National Institute of Allergy and Infectious Diseases, and others are exploring substances that might stimulate a patient's cells to manufacture more interferon than they otherwise would. These substances are known as interferon inducers.

The first interferon-inducing drug experimentally employed in humans was a substance called pyran copolymer. While it did stimulate cells to produce interferon, Stanford's Dr. Merigan, who conducted the tests, also found it to have significant undesirable side effects, and development was discontinued.

Another drug, poly I:C, was demonstrated to be a good interferon inducer in early animal trials, but when it was employed in humans the response was found to be unreliable. In addition, among its numerous undesirable side effects was a particularly serious one: hyporeactivity. It seems that after repeated dosages, interferon production by cells actually decreases, which is just the opposite of what we want to happen. Work on poly I:C continued, however, and an improved version—a drug called poly IC:LC—was developed at the National Institutes of Health.

Dr. Levy reported encouraging results with poly IC:LC in test animals, including primates. The drug proved to be a more powerful interferon inducer than its predecessor, and although side effects were observed, they were less pronounced and very short-lived. The greater potency of poly IC:LC means lower dosages and less severity of side effects and hyporeactivity. Studies are currently under way to determine the minimum dosages needed to be effective; once they are completed, human trials will be conducted. The disease against which use of poly IC:LC is contemplated is herpes encephalitis.

A FINAL NOTE

"Futurehope" is an appropriate title not only for this chapter but for the new age of antiviral drug research in which we are now living. The altruistic and commercial motivation to find safe and effective treatment agents for herpes and other viral diseases is great. It is certainly sufficient to have spurred activity in government research institutions, academic research laboratories, and pharmaceutical research-and-development operations—in short, every scientific quarter to whom we traditionally turn for help.

What will tomorrow be like? Certainly some of the drugs being worked on today will disappear as different and better ones are discovered. Several new substances are in development right now, but the work is at the preliminary stage. And certainly some of the substances that are presently available will be made more effective and safer as new approaches to using them are developed. Iontophoresis is already being tested as a way to achieve better tissue penetration by topical ara-A. So is another technique, combination therapy, which is being studied as a means of achieving greater effectiveness with antiviral compounds used internally. It looks as though drugs used in combination with each other at very low dosages can lead to an effect called therapeutic synergy, in which the action of one drug enhances the action of the others far beyond the effect that could be achieved by using any one of them alone; greater safety is also a factor.

Just ten years ago antiviral agents were a dream. Now they are a reality. No fewer than half a dozen agents have been developed for the treatment of herpes; two have already been licensed for use in the United States and the rest are under intensive study. And although there are problems with all of them, these problems are not considered to be insurmountable and they will all ultimately be solved. The speed with which tomorrow is approaching is staggering. In fact, many scientists believe tomorrow has already arrived, and certainly, as we have seen, insofar as treating herpes keratitis and herpes encephalitis is concerned, Futurehope is now.

CHAPTER 12

NOW THAT YOU KNOW: MORE QUESTIONS

Here we are, at what I had originally planned as the end of a penetrating, interesting, useful, and comprehensive look at herpes simplex, one of the most widespread viral illnesses to affect humankind, and at the many things people can do to help themselves cope with it. But is it the end? Have I really covered it all?

As I prepared to bring my survey to a close, I realized that I had overlooked one crucial factor: the more you learn, the more you want to learn. Answers not only satisfy a fundamental need to know but, if they are good answers, they invariably spawn new questions, better questions, questions you would only think of asking once you knew something about the subject.

A new ending began to take shape and finally emerged as this final chapter, which contains the myriad questions typically asked by patients in the know.

In addition to answering questions that reflect an advanced level of curiosity and interest, we will identify additional resources that are available to anyone who wants to know more, become more involved, or simply keep abreast

174

of the research developments as they are reported. This is perhaps the only way a book on herpes can end—at the beginning.

And now, let's go one step beyond.

Q.   Let's say two people in a relationship both have herpes. If they don't practice prevention, can they reinfect each other? And, if they can, does it make a difference in their experience of herpes?

A.   First, they definitely can reinfect each other. Having herpes doesn't protect you from contracting more of the same viruses if exposed because, unlike other infections, herpes does not confer the host with complete immunity. In fact, having herpes doesn't even protect you entirely from the threat of your own herpes simplex viruses; for this reason, autoinoculation is a potential problem we have to prevent.

The significance of reinfection is not apparent at this time, but the introduction of more viruses into the body is undesirable in any case. If you have labial herpes and contract genital herpes from your partner, you now have an additional site where annoying recurrences may crop up. If you are a woman, you will now have to take PAP tests more frequently than would otherwise be necessary. Should you become pregnant, you must take precautions against infecting your newborn, a fully preventable situation but one you would not be confronted with if you hadn't become infected genitally.

The answer to the question of reinfection becomes still less apparent when both people have the infection at the same site, genitally or orally. Some scientists speculate that the introduction of additional herpes simplex viruses increases the chances for recurrence, since the number of cells that harbor the latent virus is likely to be greater. Other scientists say that the number of viruses produced during an active outbreak is so great that more wouldn't make any difference. Both postulates are reasonable, and the issue is further clouded by couples in my own practice—and the practice of other physicians with whom I have spoken—who report that they have ceased all attempts at prevention with no ill effects.

Without any scientific evidence to guide us, it almost becomes a matter of opinion. My personal judgment would be to practice prevention until the issue is better defined. I'd hate to find out too late that more viruses do indeed make matters worse.

Q. I read somewhere that men might be able to transmit genital herpes without having sores, which contradicts what you said earlier about transmission being possible only during active outbreaks. Is there any truth to this?

A. What you probably read was the University of Florida School of Medicine's seven-year-old report indicating that HSV had been isolated from the urogenital tracts of men who had no history of herpes. Before we reach any premature conclusions, let's take a look at the facts.

In 1973, cultures were taken from the urethras and prostate glands of a group of 263 men with a variety of urologic problems. The herpes simplex virus was recovered from the urogenital tracts of thirty-nine of the men (15 percent of the total) despite the fact that none had external sores or, to their knowledge, any history of herpes. To say the least, this was an unexpected and frightening report that seemed to defy what we thought we knew about herpes. Immediately, investigators throughout the country began studies to validate those findings.

None was successful. After six years, no investigator was able to culture HSV from the urethras of men with or without a prior history of herpes. In fact, at the very same institution from which the first results were reported, attempts to reproduce those findings ended in failure.

Scientists cannot explain those first results; the only possible explanation is that some statistical fluke concentrated an extremely rare biologic event (viral shedding without active infection) into one study at one time. The fact that the findings couldn't be reproduced in tests on thousands of men nationwide allayed most scientists' fears that this was a problem. If anything, it is so rare and so insignificant that it isn't worth worrying about. The standard view of transmission has not changed: no prodrome or sores, no worry.

Q.   Have researchers ever found a connection between labial, facial, or oral herpes and cancer of the lip, mouth, or throat?

A.   At a seminar sponsored by the American Cancer Society in St. Augustine, Florida, in April 1974, Dr. Albert Sabin reported finding HSV antibodies among 183 patients suffering from fourteen different kinds of cancer, including cancer of the skin, lips, larynx, kidney, prostate, and cervix. Dr. Sabin also reported that he was unable to find HSV antibodies among 175 other patients with cancer of the lung, breast, or stomach.

Another physician, Dr. Ariel Hollinshead of George Washington University, found HSV antibodies in the blood of 90 percent of patients suffering from head and neck tumors called squamous cell carcinomas. These findings, however, were clouded by the fact that most of these patients were heavy smokers; the cancers may have been the result of heavy smoking, not HSV.

Dr. Fred Rapp of the Pennsylvania State University School of Medicine has demonstrated that both HSV-1 and HSV-2 can transform normal hamster cells into cancer cells, and, as we have learned, HSV-1 is still most frequently associated with labial herpes. These findings signify that cellular defects can be caused by either HSV-1 or HSV-2 in either lip or cervical cells. But keep in mind that an association has been made between genital herpes and cancer of the cervix, not between labial herpes and cancer. So far, no investigator has established a firm connection between labial, facial, or oral herpes and any form of cancer.

Q. Has any connection ever been made between genital herpes and some cancers in males?

A. Not really. It is true that, in theory, cellular defects caused by a virus like HSV can occur in any tissue affected by the virus, regardless of the sex of the host. Since the incidence of genital herpes is quite evenly divided between males and females, it would seem logical to expect infected males to run a greater risk of urogenital cancers, just as females do with respect to cervical cancer, and to encounter the same statistical certainty demonstrated by cervical cancer data. In reality, however, no one has been able to make that association in men.

The data that Dr. Albert Sabin presented at the American Cancer Society seminar in 1974 were highly inconclusive. The total number of males who were found to have both urogenital cancer and HSV antibodies was tiny and could easily be explained by coincidence. The same is true of Dr. Centifanto's data from the

University of Florida School of Medicine; some men with urogenital cancer were also found to have genital herpes, but, again, coincidence easily explains the findings.

In response to the objection that the reason a possible relationship between genital herpes and male urogenital cancer hasn't been found is because it hasn't been studied as intensely as cervical cancer, I can only say that the relationship between genital herpes and cervical cancer jumped out at scientists. The data were so compelling and so indicative that subsequent studies merely served to better define what was obvious from the beginning. There are no such indications of any kind to motivate scientists to search for a possible HSV link to male cancers. To conduct intensive studies that would merely confirm the lack of a relationship would be a waste of scarce research resources.

At present, no connection has been found between genital herpes in men and urogenital cancer.

Q. Is there any relationship between genital herpes in men and impotence?

A. Yes, but it is a psychological rather than a physical aspect of the disease. Impotence in herpes patients stems from two basic fears: fear of spreading herpes and fear of rejection because of herpes. While my practice may not be representative of what other physicians see (I have many herpes patients), my general impression is that impotence related to herpes is more common than most people realize. Fortunately, however, it is short-lived and can easily be reversed by counseling.

A strong reluctance to spread the virus to anyone else is common among people with herpes, particularly genital herpes, and it runs deep. Of all the patients with various infectious diseases I have treated, herpes patients are unique in having this pronounced feeling. When this feeling becomes fear, it can lead to many forms of dysfunctional behavior, including social withdrawal, a lack of interest in sex, and, in some men, impotence. When the desire not to spread herpes is channeled productively and motivates preventive behavior, however, the fear loses its force to precipitate dysfunctions, including impotence.

The fear of being rejected because of herpes can also lead to dysfunctional behavior. Social withdrawal appears to be most common, but I have seen patients whose sexual performance has been hampered as well. While it is true that some patients have psychological problems that run far deeper than and predate those sparked by herpes, I am constantly amazed at how many previously well-adjusted, outgoing, generally happy patients develop a fear of rejection after contracting genital herpes. Much of this fear dissipates upon learning about the disease and getting into a wellness orientation, but sometimes the patient may feel a need for professional counseling.

While we are on this subject, let me share a corollary observation I have made. Many patients who overcome their fears and adjust to having herpes still have difficulty relating to other people. They aren't afraid of spreading the disease because they know how to prevent it, and they aren't afraid of being rejected. They simply don't know how to communicate the fact that they have herpes, and they know that how they talk about it will influence the attitude of the other person. This can be a big problem for a single person. Let's explore some possible solutions with the next question.

Q. When, why, and how should I tell another person that I have herpes?

A. Let's establish some ground rules before answering this question. First, your concern shouldn't pertain to labial herpes; I have yet to treat a patient or meet anyone whose relationships with other people have been complicated by lip herpes. Second, this question applies only to single people. Third, we define "another person" as a potential sex partner.

Now, let's reconstruct the question and pose it in a more direct way: How do I tell a prospective sex partner about genital herpes in a manner that doesn't frighten him or her away? Let's impose one more constraint as we develop an answer. The person you want to tell is someone you intend to see over a period of time; otherwise, why bother telling him or her at all? If you are not infectious at the time of a casual sexual encounter, the fact that you have herpes is irrelevant.

Now, why is telling that other person necessary? I can think of two reasons. (1) At some point in your relationship, you might have a recurrence and have to practice prevention— that is, abstain from sex. If sex is a normal part of your relationship, you will want the understanding, support, and encouragement of the other person during this period. (2) There is a possibility that, despite your best efforts to prevent it, the other person may become infected. It does occasionally happen, and your partner has a right to know about this possibility in advance.

My advice about *how* to let another person know you have herpes is to do so privately, calmly, directly (without any introductory fanfare like, "I have this big secret to tell you" or "There's something about me I think you should know"), and in a nonthreatening way. You might start with a simple question like, "Have you ever heard of herpes?" or, perhaps even better, "Do you know what cold sores are?" and take it from there. Talk about cold sores, which are neutral; most people know what they are and aren't frightened by them. Draw the parallel between labial herpes and genital herpes. Don't harp on how terrible herpes can be: talk about how relatively insignificant a problem it is. Avoid the word "incurable." Instead, explain that the disease is self-limiting, although sometimes it can recur, just like chickenpox. Keep in mind that a lot of myths surround herpes, so stick to the facts— for, as we know, the facts aren't all that bad. Talk about how easy it is to prevent herpes, and how when two people cooperate the chances of spreading it are almost nil. If the situation warrants it, ask the other person to read this book.

I can honestly say that I have never seen a properly conducted conversation about herpes bring a relationship to an end. I do know some herpes patients who frightened their partners so thoroughly that the latter understandably wanted no part of the relationship, but I attribute this to the way the information was presented. These same patients had far better results their next time around.

One possibility that you may encounter when you try to tell other people about herpes is that they already know about it. Since herpes is so widespread, the person you tell may also have the infection and know a great deal about the subject. Or, if that person does have herpes but doesn't know much about it, you may be able to furnish the missing facts and help in a big way.

Q.   Can a person who doesn't have herpes do anything to prevent getting it?

A.   There are a few things a person without herpes can do to avoid it, but, in the main, prevention is the responsibility of those who are infected. Here are some helpful tips.

Don't kiss a person who has a cold sore. If you do so inadvertently, wash your lips with soap and water immediately.

Don't share a drinking glass or eating utensils with a person who has a cold sore.

As unromantic as it sounds, ask new sex partners if they have genital herpes. While some may react negatively to such a question, many won't, considering the growing awareness of the magnitude of this infection.

Equally unromantic and often impractical, don't be afraid to inspect the genitals of a new sex partner. If you notice a sore or cluster of sores, it might be herpes.

If you are a male, always use a condom; if you are a female, always insist that a new sex partner use one.

While these tips may prove helpful in some situations, an uninfected person can always protect him or herself by understanding, supporting, and encouraging the preventive behavior of those who are infected.

Q.   I heard somewhere that recurrences have been related to the menstrual cycle. Is this true?

A.   Not generally. Some women have reported a pattern of recurrence that correlates with their menstrual cycle, and the hormonal shifts that occur at this time may be a factor—but this situation is rare. Dr. Lawrence Corey of the University of Washington and others have conducted numerous studies of recurrence patterns and rates in which hundreds of women and thousands of recurrent episodes have been analyzed. Menstruation has never appeared as a link. So while it can happen and, according to some women, has happened, menstruation seems to be quite unrelated to recurrences.

Q. Are venereal warts and genital herpes related?

A. No. The only things venereal warts have in common with genital herpes is that both are caused by viruses, although the viruses are unrelated, and both are transmitted by sexual contact.

Venereal warts are caused by the papova group of viruses and appear as small growths on the surface of skin or mucosal tissue. They don't come and go as do herpes sores and they don't typically hurt as does herpes when it is active. Venereal warts can be treated with a number of dissolving chemicals or they can be removed by freezing, burning, or surgical excision.

Q. Is there any similarity between herpes and VD?

A. Technically, genital herpes is a form of VD, as is labial herpes among people who practice oral sexual relations. Since the term VD is being replaced by the more accurate term STD (for "sexually transmissible diseases"), there's no question that herpes fits in.

But other than sharing a similar mode of transmission, herpes and most forms of STD differ in a fundamental regard: although herpes can't be cured, it only rarely leads to serious complications, whereas untreated syphilis, gonorrhea, and nongonococcal urethritis (NGU) —the most commonly transmitted sex-related diseases today—almost always do. Without treatment, syphilis can lead to blindness, insanity, paralysis, and death; untreated gonorrhea and NGU can lead to chronic pelvic inflammatory disease in women, which in turn can result in fallopian-tube damage and sterility. In men, untreated NGU can cause epididymitis, a potentially sterilizing infection of the tube through which sperm must flow.

In terms of potential complications that can result, herpes is considerably less serious than these other common infections.

Q. Has anyone ever studied the long-term effect of herpes on the nerve tissue in which the latent virus resides?

A. To date there have been no well-controlled, scientific, longitudinal studies of genital or labial herpes patients. However, many herpes patients have been followed clinically over many years, so there is some information.

Many of the studies concerning treatment agents, cervical cancer, and the natural course of the disease that we have reviewed, particularly the better ones in which random patient selection procedures were employed, have included subjects aged 50 to 80 with histories of infection spanning twenty to fifty years. Although the length of infection has never been the specific focus of these or other studies, researchers have noted that the constellation of symptoms and problems observed in long-term patients does not differ from that observed in patients with new or relatively short-term infections.

While no one can state with absolute certainty that herpes does not affect nerve tissue, there is not one shred of evidence that it does. The current view on the subject is that when nerve cells harbor the latent form of HSV-1 or HSV-2, no replication takes place at all. Viral degeneration of nerve tissue or viral interference with nerve function is not known to occur.

Q. Where can I have herpes diagnosed?

A. As we learned earlier, the diagnosis of herpes is not a particularly complex problem. Most of the time, the symptoms are so classical and their pattern of appearance so characteristic that any astute physician can make a clinical diagnosis of herpes and be right more than 90 percent of the time. Of course, the clinical orientation of the doctor makes a difference in how experienced and familiar he or she is with herpes, and therefore gynecologists, dermatologists, urologists, internists, family practitioners, and general practitioners are most likely to be well equipped to make a clinical diagnosis. Physicians who practice in VD clinics can also diagnose herpes clinically, because they see great numbers of patients with urogenital and oralpharyngeal complaints and are quite adept at sorting out the symptoms.

In cases where clinical diagnosis proves inconclusive, there are a variety of laboratory tests that will provide more definition, the most accurate of which is the tissue culture. Unfortunately, the tissue culture is the least accessible of all the diagnostic tests for herpes because most labs have neither the equipment nor the systems necessary to perform it. However, tissue-culture systems are maintained by most state public-health laboratories and most medical schools. Your doctor may decide to refer you to one of these places or make special arrangements to send the specimen to the nearest lab capable of handling it.

Q. Is herpes an important public priority?

A. I would have to say no, at least not yet. Despite the fact that most public-health officials, medical administrators, and government health policymakers clearly recognize that herpes is an ever-growing major epidemic, they generally regard it as a nuisance condition with no serious consequences; in addition, they often feel that any attempt at control would be relatively ineffective. Thus herpes prevention, education, and control receive virtually no attention or government backing, and research receives minimal support. I personally feel that this view is not balanced and take exception to it.

While herpes is not the life-threatening health issue that cancer, heart disease, or stroke is, it can affect the psychological health of millions of Americans, serve as a complicating factor in a number of medical conditions such as cancer and organ transplantation, and directly result in serious, though infrequent, complications such as brain damage, loss of vision, and infant mortality. Technological barriers make it impractical to employ such traditional epidemic-control strategies as mass immunization or mass screening and treatment, but potentially effective nonmedical control approaches—public information and education programs—haven't even been tried. A problem as widespread as herpes should become a major public issue.

Research is the only area where some governmental interest and support are evident, but even here herpes has low priority. In striking a balance between the magnitude and severity of a problem and the amount of resources allocated to finding a solution, I believe herpes research comes up short. Of the $3.5 billion annually invested by government in biomedical research, cancer consumes $1 billion, heart disease $500 million, and neurological disorders (including stroke) $250 million. The amount going to herpes research is between $2 and $4 million a year—not an insignificant amount, but not really enough in terms of existing research needs.

Q. What can the average person do to help?

A. Use the available outlets for influencing elected representatives and government officials who develop public policy. To illustrate, let me tell you how I have used such outlets.

I have written letters to my senators and congressional representatives informing them that I consider herpes to be a major public-health issue that is not being adequately addressed by government. I called on them to generate public initiatives to solve the herpes problem and emphasized that I would support their efforts.

I have written to the Secretary of Health, Education, and Welfare and the Surgeon General of the U.S. Public Health Service asking them to exercise greater executive leadership and direction in the search for cures and vaccines for herpes.

Whenever I read an article about herpes in a newspaper or magazine, I write a laudatory letter to the editor and call for more such articles and more public discussion about this issue in the print media.

Whenever I hear a radio or television broadcast about herpes, I write the station manager and voice my support for such programing.

Now, I'm not naive—I realize that isolated letters here and there have only limited impact on the formation of public policy. Surely a broad-based constituency for increased government interest in herpes would be a thousand times more effective, but I feel that something is better than nothing. I believe that herpes receives so little attention not because it is actively opposed politically but because the issue is submerged. Even a handful of letters might stimulate some curiosity or provide a slightly different context for policymaking.

I would encourage you to do as I have done. Voice your concerns and interests to your elected representatives and government officials, and support greater discussion of the issue in the print and electronic media. After all, public policy does reflect what the public feels is important. Let the people who have to gauge public sentiment know what you think.

Q. What *about* a broad-based constituency? Are there any interest groups concerned with herpes as there are for cancer, multiple sclerosis, diabetes, or birth defects?

A. As a matter of fact, there is one—the American Social Health Association, a voluntary health organization. It is a tax-exempt nonprofit agency that, among other things, works toward ensuring that government priorities reflect its special interests—in this case, chiefly herpes and several other direct-contact diseases.

Members and staff work directly with congressional representatives, senators, and administrative officials on pertinent legislation and budgetary issues that could affect herpes research and prevention programs. They also testify at congressional hearings on health and research needs and generally keep the focus on herpes alive with periodic "issue papers" and other reports. But they are perhaps most important and effective in coordinating the activities of a broad, grass-roots constituency who favor greater government response to the herpes problem.

The American Social Health Association has a nationwide membership of over 15,000 people who receive regular newsletters and special reports and who, when a show of force and popular support is needed, are asked to participate in massive letter-writing campaigns. I have taken part in several of these efforts and can tell you that they are quite effective. If you are politically inclined and want to get involved, get in touch with them at the following address: American Social Health Association, 260 Sheridan Avenue, Palo Alto, CA 94306. Membership costs are $8.00 per year and are tax-deductible.

Q. You mentioned that the American Social Health Association does other things besides influence government policy. What else does it do that is specifically related to herpes?

A. It supports the biomedical research of scientists who are looking for solutions to the herpes problem, and it furnishes a special service to people with herpes who want to know about the latest scientific developments as they happen.

The research program of the American Social Health Association is targeted to provide seed money to scientists and medical investigators so that new approaches or innovative ideas can be nurtured and developed to the point where they can qualify for much larger federal research grants. It is financed entirely by private contributions and is one of the only research programs that channel every dollar into research without an overhead charge (most research funds take 10 to 30 percent for administrative expenses, leaving only seventy to ninety cents out of every dollar raised for actual research).

The special service for people who have herpes is called HELP (it's not an acronym, it's just HELP), and for the $8.00 annual membership fee you receive four issues (one every twelve weeks) of a journal that covers every aspect of herpes. The journal contains research reports, suggestions about how to cope with herpes, and answers to questions sent in by subscribers.

In addition, subscribers are given the

opportunity to participate in nationwide survey-research projects, attend seminars about herpes conducted throughout the country, and become part of local discussion groups in which people with herpes can meet each other and share information and common concerns. Many doctors subscribe to this service, for the journal is the only publication of its kind that continually keeps abreast of scientific developments and progress in herpes research.

If the HELP service sounds worthwhile and interesting, you can join by writing the American Social Health Association at the address given above, to the attention of HELP.

Q. Can I participate in herpes research projects, and, if so, how?

A. This is one of the questions most frequently asked by patients. Interest in taking part in clinical trials of new antiviral treatment agents runs high. Almost anyone can enroll in a herpes experiment, but before you do so, consider the following points.

First, since most herpes research is conducted at medical centers associated with medical schools, you must live near one in order for your participation to be practical for both you and the researchers. Follow-up is an essential part of a study, and most investigators aren't interested in subjects who can't return on a regular basis. (Enough "loss to follow-up," as it is called, invalidates a study.)

Second, you have to make certain that the institution near you conducts herpes research, which you can find out through the HELP service or by calling the various departments most likely to be engaging in such research— for example, virology, infectious disease, dermatology, gynecology, and medicine.

Third, you have to fit into the needs of the

study. Sometimes only males are wanted, sometimes only females, or some research calls only for genital herpes patients or for labial herpes patients.

Finally, and this is the qualification most patients have trouble accepting because everyone wants to receive the promising drug being tested, if the study employs placebo controls, you will have no say as to whether you are assigned to the test group or the control group. But take heart—if the drug is found to be effective, everyone who constituted the placebo group will be called back to receive the real drug.

Q.   Before reading this book, I thought herpes was far more fearsome, serious, and complicated. Now it almost sounds like a "piece of cake." Is my changed attitude too good to be true?

A.   I don't think so. Before reading this book, your thoughts—and indeed most people's thoughts about herpes—were probably a collection of incomplete ideas founded on myth, misinformation, and isolated exaggerations of certain aspects of the disease, you now have a broad perspective based on fact. You are less fearful because the objective realities about herpes don't warrant fear; you are less worried about how serious and complicated herpes can be because you have learned how infrequently difficulties arise and how most of them can be prevented by your informed actions.

In the introduction to this book, I stated that insofar as herpes is concerned knowledge is power and hope; your changed attitude bears out this contention. The great fear of the unknown, compounded by misapprehension and mistaken views, has been replaced by factual insights and a balanced appreciation of how manageable herpes is; you have the power and hope to achieve wellness and lead a complete and productive life unencumbered by this disease. Far from being too good to be true, your changed attitude is most appropriate and natural, considering how much you now know.

My final hope is that the interest and thirst for information whetted by this book will give rise to more questions, more discussion, more demands for research, and a new public and private health perspective on herpes.

REFERENCES

Ader, R., and Cohen, N. "Behaviorally Conditioned Immunosuppression." *Psychosomatic Medicine* 37 (1975): 333–340.

Akins, W. R., and Nurnberg, G. *How to Meditate Without Attending a TM Class.* New York: Amjon, 1976.

Anderson, T. W. "Large-Scale Trials of Vitamin C." *Annals of the New York Academy of Science* 258 (1975):498.

Anderson, T. W., Reid, D. W. W., and Beaton, G. H. "Vitamin C and the Common Cold: A Double-Blind Trial." *Journal of the Canadian Medical Association* 107 (1972):503.

Anderson, F. D., Ushijima, R. N., and Larson, C. L. "Recurrent Herpes Genitalis Treatment with Mycobacterium Bovis (BCG)." *Journal of Obstetrics and Gynecology* 43 (1974):797–805.

Antonovsky, A. *Health, Stress, and Coping.* San Francisco: Jossey-Bass, 1979.

Baringer, J. R. "Recovery of Herpes Simplex Virus from Human Sacral Ganglions." *New England Journal of Medicine* 291 (1974):828–830.

Baringer, J. R., and Swoveland, P. "Recovery of Herpes Simplex Virus from Human Trigeminal Ganglions." *New England Journal of Medicine* 291 (1974):648–650.

Bathrop, R. W. "Depressed Lymphocyte Function After Bereavement." *The Lancet* 1 (1977):834–836.

Benson, H. "Your Innate Asset for Combating Stress." *Harvard Business Review* 52 (1974):49–60.

_____. *The Relaxation Response.* New York: William Morrow, 1975.

Bierman, S. M. "BCG Immunoprophylaxis of Recurrent Herpes ProGenitalis." *Archives of Dermatology* 112 (1976):1410–1415.

_____. "The Mechanism of Recurrent Infection by Herpes Virus Hominis." *Archives of Dermatology* 112 (1976): 1459–1461.

Blank, H., and Brody, M. W. "Recurrent Herpes Simplex: A Psychiatric and Laboratory Study." *Psychosomatic Medicine* 12 (1950):254–260.

Blough, H. A., and Giuntoli, R. L. "Successful Treatment of Human Genital Herpes Infections with 2-Deoxy-d-glucose." *Journal of the American Medical Association* 241 (1979):2798–2801.

Bourne, G. H. "Vitamin C and Immunity." *British Journal of Nutrition* 2 (1949):341.

Brown, B. *New Mind, New Body.* New York: Harper & Row, 1975.

Callahan, J. "The Herpes Epidemic." *New Times,* June 12, 1978.

Canter, A., Imboden, J. B., and Cluff, L. E. "The Frequency of Physical Illness and a Function of Prior Vulnerability and Contemporary Stress." *Psychosomatic Medicine* 28 (1966):344–350.

Carter, W. A., ed. *Selective Inhibitors of Viral Functions.* Cleveland: C.R.C. Press, 1973.

Centifanto, Y. M., Drylie, D. M., Deardourff, S. L., et al. "Herpes Virus Type 2 in the Male Genitourinary Tract." *Science* 178 (1972):318–319.

Corey, L., Reeves, W. C., Chiang, W. T., et al. "Ineffectiveness of Topical Ether for the Treatment of Genital Herpes Virus Infection." *New England Journal of Medicine* 299 (1978):237–239.

Corey, L., Reeves, W. C., and Holmes, K. K. "Cellular Immune Response in Genital Herpes Simplex Virus Infection." *New England Journal of Medicine* 299 (1978):986–991.

Corey, L., Stamm, W., Reeves, W. C., et al. "Controlled Trial of BCG Vaccine for the Prevention of Recurrent Genital Herpes." Abstract, 16th Interscience Conference on Antimicrobial Agents and Chemotherapy.

Danziger, S. "Ice Packs for Cold Sores." *The Lancet* 1 (1978): 103.

Deutsch, R. M. *Realities of Nutrition.* Palo Alto, Calif.: Bull, 1976.

Douglas, R. G. Jr., and Couch, R. B. "A Prospective Study of Chronic Herpes Simplex Virus Infection and Recurrent Herpes Labialis in Humans." *Journal of Immunology* 104 (1970):289–295.

"Dye-Light Therapy for Herpes Simplex?" *Medical World News,* February 22, 1974, pp. 39–55.

Finter, N. B., ed. *Interferon and Interferon Inducers.* New York: Elsevier, 1973.

Frankel-Conrat, H. *Design and Function at the Threshold of Life: The Viruses.* New York: Academic Press, 1962.

Glasser, R. *The Body Is Hero.* New York: Random House, 1976.

Gold, E., and Nankervis, G. A. In A. S. Kaplan, ed., *The Herpes Viruses.* New York: Academic Press, 1973.

Griffith, R. S., Norins, A. L., and Kagan, C. "A Multicentered Study of Lysine Therapy in Herpes Simplex Infection." *Dermatologica* 156 (1978):257–267.

Hanshaw, J. B. "Herpes Virus Hominis Infections in the Fetus and the Newborn." *American Journal of Diseases of Children* 126 (1973):546–555.

"Herpes Patients Fight Medicine's Empty Cupboard." *Medical World News,* July 23, 1979, pp. 27–28.

Hinkle, L. E. Jr. "The Effects of Exposure to Cultural Change, Social Change, and Changes in Interpersonal Relationships on Health." In B. S. Dohrenwend and B. P. Dohrenwend, eds., *Stressful Life Events: Their Nature and Effects.* New York: Wiley, 1974.

Hollinshead, A. C., and Knaus, W. A. "Herpes Viruses—A Link in the Cancer Chain?" *Chemistry* 50 (1977):17–21.

Holmes, T. H., and Rahe, R. H. "The Social Readjustment Rating Scale." *Journal of Psychosomatic Research* 11 (1967):213–218.

Jacobson, L. *You Must Relax.* New York: McGraw-Hill, 1962.

Juel-Jensen, B. E., and MacCallum, F. O. *Herpes Simplex, Varicella, and Zoster.* Philadelphia: J. B. Lippincott, 1972.

Kagan, J. "Herpes: It Can Be Treated—But Not Cured." *Ms.* magazine, January 1978.

Kaslow, A. L., and Miles, R. B., *Freedom from Chronic Disease.* Los Angeles: J. P. Tarcher, 1979.

Kennaway, E. L. "The Racial and Social Incidence of Cancer of the Uterus." *British Journal of Cancer* 2 (1948):176–212.

Kern, A. B., and Schiff, B. L. "Vaccine Therapy in Recurrent Herpes Simplex." *Archives of Dermatology* 89 (1964):844–845.

_____. "Smallpox Vaccinations in the Management of Recurrent Herpes Simplex: A Controlled Evaluation." *Journal of Investigative Dermatology* 89 (1964): 844–845.

Korsager, B., Spence, E. S., Nordhorst, C. H., et al. "Herpes Virus Hominis Infections in Renal Transplant Recipients." *Scandinavian Journal of Infectious Diseases* 7 (1975):11–19.

Larsen, J. W. Jr., and Grossman, J. H. III. "Genital Herpes Virus During Pregnancy." *Perinatal Infection Newsletter* 1 (1978):1–4.

Lazarus, R. S. *Psychological Stress and the Coping Process.* New York: McGraw-Hill, 1966.

Marks, R. G. "New Hope in Herpes Genitalis?" *Current Prescribing,* March 1979.

Maugh, T. H. II. "Chemotherapy: Antiviral Agents Come of Age." *Science* 192 (1976):128–132.

"Medical News: Promising New Antiherpes Agent Being Tested in Humans." *Journal of the American Medical Association* 240 (1978):2231–2232.

Merigan, T. C. "Host Defense Against Virus Infections." *New England Journal of Medicine* 290 (1974):323–329.

————, ed. *Antivirals with Clinical Potential.* Chicago: University of Chicago Press, 1976.

Miller, J. B. "Treatment of Active Herpes Virus Infections with Influenza Virus Vaccine." *Annals of Allergy* 42 (1979):295–305.

Milman, N., Scheibel, J., and Jessen, O. "Failure of Lysine Treatment in Recurring Herpes Simplex Labialis." *The Lancet* 2 (1978):942.

Montgomerie, J. Z., Becroft, D. M., Croxson, M. C., et al. "Herpes Simplex Virus Infections in Renal Transplant Recipients." *The Lancet* 2 (1969):867–871.

Myers, M. G., Oxman, M. N., Clark, J. E., et al. "Failure of Neutral-Red Photodynamic Inactivation in Recurrent Herpes Simplex Virus Infections." *New England Journal of Medicine* 293 (1975):945–949.

Nahmias, A. J., Alford, C. A., and Korones, S. B. "Infection of the Newborn with Herpes Virus Hominis." *Advances in Pediatrics* 17 (1970):185–226.

Nahmias, A. J., and Roizman, B. "Infection with Herpes-Simplex Viruses 1 and 2." *New England Journal of Medicine* 289 (1973):667–674, 719–724, 781–789.

Nahmias, A. J., Naib, Z. M., and Josey, W. E. "Epidemiological Studies Relating Genital Herpetic Infection to Cervical Carcinoma." *Cancer Research* 34 (1974):1111–1117.

————. "Antibodies to Herpes Virus Hominis Type 1 and 2 in Humans: Patients with Genital Herpetic Infections." *American Journal of Epidemiology* 91 (1970):539–546.

————. "Significance of Herpes Simplex Virus Infection During Pregnancy." *Clinical Obstetrics and Gynecology* 15 (1971):929–938.

National Institute of Allergy and Infectious Diseases. Virology Task Force Report. U.S. Department of Health, Education, and Welfare, Public Health Service, National Institutes of Health, Washington, D.C.: 1979.

Notkins, A. L. "Immune Mechanisms by Which the Spread of Viral Infections Is Stopped." *Cell Immunology* 11 (1974):478–483.

Overall, J. C. Jr. "Dermatologic Diseases." In G. J. Galasso, T. C. Merigan, and R. A. Buchanan, eds. *Antiviral Agents and*

Viral Diseases of Man. New York: Raven Press, 1979.

Parker, J. D. "A Double-Blind Trial of Idoxuridine in Recurrent Genital Herpes." In J. S. Oxford, F. A. Drasar, and J. D. Williams, eds., *Chemotherapy of Herpes Simplex Virus Infection.* London: Academic Press, 1972.

Pasricha, J. S., Nayyar, K. C., and Pasricha, A. "A New Method for Treatment of Herpes Simplex." *Archives of Dermatology* 107 (1973):775.

Pauling, L. *Vitamin C and the Common Cold.* San Francisco: W. H. Freeman, 1970.

Pelletier, K. R. *Mind as Healer, Mind as Slayer.* New York: Delta, 1977.

Rapp, F. "Herpes Viruses, Venereal Disease, and Cancer." *American Scientist* 66 (1978):670–674.

Rapp, F., and Reed, C. "Experimental Evidence for the Oncogenic Potential of Herpes Simplex Virus." *Cancer Research* 36 (1976):800–806.

Rattray, M. C., Corey, L., Reeves, W. C., et al. "Recurrent Genital Herpes Among Women: Symptomatic vs. Asymptomatic Viral Shedding." *British Journal of Venereal Diseases* 54 (1978):262–265.

Rawls, W. E., Gardner, H. L., Flanders, R. W., et al. "Genital Herpes in Two Social Groups." *American Journal of Obstetrics and Gynecology* 110 (1971):682–689.

Rawls, W. E., Tompkins, W. A. F., and Melnick, S. L. "The Association of Herpes Virus Type 2 and Carcinoma of the Uterine Cervix." *American Journal of Epidemiology* 89 (1969):547.

Reuben, D. *Everything You Always Wanted to Know About Nutrition.* New York: Simon and Schuster, 1978.

———. "The Grim New Venereal Disease in Our Midst." *Reader's Digest,* November 1974.

Roizman, B. "Herpes Viruses, Man, and Cancer—Or the Persistence of the Viruses of Love." In J. Monod and E. Borek, eds., *Of Microbes and Life.* New York: Columbia University Press, 1971.

Rosenfeld, A. "Provocative Talk at an Interferon Workshop." *Life,* July 1979.

Rosenberg, G. L., Snyderman, R., and Notkins, A. L. "Production of Chemotactic Factors and Lymphokines in Human Leukocytes Stimulated with Herpes Simplex Virus." *Infection and Immunity* 10 (1974):111–115.

Russell, A. S. "Cell-Mediated Immunity to Herpes Simplex Virus in Man." *American Journal of Clinical Pathology* 60 (1973):826–830.

Sabin, A. B. "Misery of Recurrent Herpes: What to Do?" *New England Journal of Medicine* 293 (1973):986–988.

Samuels, M., and Bennett, H. *Be Well.* New York: Random House, 1974.

Schneck, J. M. "The Psychological Component in a Case of Herpes Simplex." *Psychosomatic Medicine* 9 (1947):62–64.

Selye, H. *The Stress of Life.* New York: McGraw-Hill, 1956.

———. *Stress Without Distress.* New York: J. B. Lippincott, 1974.

Shealy, N. *90 Days to Self-Health.* New York: Dial Press, 1977.

Shipkowitz, N. L., Bower, R. R., and Appel, R. N. "Suppression of Herpes Simplex Virus Infection by Phosphoacetic Acid." *Applied Microbiology* 26 (1973):264–276.

Simonton, O. C., Matthews-Simonton, S., and Creighton, J. *Getting Well Again.* Los Angeles: J. P. Tarcher, 1978.

Subak-Sharpe, G. "The Venereal Disease of the New Morality." *Today's Health,* March 1975.

Tankersley, R. W. Jr. "Amino Acid Requirements of Herpes Simplex Virus in Human Cells." *Journal of Bacteriology* 87 (1964):609–613.

Tanner, O. *Stress.* Alexandria, Va.: Time-Life Books, 1976.

Ulene, A. *Feeling Fine.* Los Angeles: J. P. Tarcher, 1977.

Underwood, E. J. *Trace Elements in Human and Animal Nutrition.* New York: Academic Press, 1971.

"Viruses and Cancer: Update." Editorial interview with Dr. Fred Rapp. *Cancer Journal for Clinicians* 28 (1978):356–361.

"Vitamin C and Immune Protection." *Science News* 115 (1979):295.

Whitley, R. J., Soong, S. J., Dolin, R., et al. "Adenine Arabinoside Therapy of Biopsy-Proved Herpes Simplex Encephalitis: NIAID Collaborative Antiviral Study." *New England Journal of Medicine* 297 (1977):289–294.

Wilton, J. M. A., Ivanyi, L., and Lehner, T. "Cell-Mediated Immunity in Herpes Virus Hominis Infections." *British Journal of Medicine* 1 (1972):723–726.

Winter, R. *Triumph Over Tension.* New York: Grosset & Dunlap, 1976.

Wise, T. G., Pavan, P. R., and Ennis, F. A. "Herpes Simplex Virus Vaccines." *Journal of Infectious Diseases* 136 (1977):706–710.

"Workshop on the Treatment and Prevention of Herpes Simplex Virus Infections." *Journal of Infectious Diseases* 277 (1973):117–119.

Zimmerman, D. R. "Self-Treatment of Cold Sores with Ice." *The Lancet* 2 (1978):1260.

INDEX

202